AMERICAN JOINT COMMITTEE ON CANCER

22082

KT-416-489

AJCC
CANCER STAGING
ATLAS

EDITORS

FREDERICK L. GREENE, M.D.
Chair, Department of General Surgery
Carolinas Medical Center
Charlotte, North Carolina

CAROLYN C. COMPTON, M.D., PH.D
Director of Biorepositories and Biospeciment Research
National Cancer Institute
Bethesda, Maryland

APRIL G. FRITZ, C.T.R., R.H.I.T.
Division of Cancer Control and Population Sciences
National Cancer Institute
Bethesda, Maryland

JATIN P. SHAH, M.D.
Chief, Head and Neck Service
Memorial Sloan-Kettering Cancer Center
New York, New York

DAVID P. WINCHESTER, M.D.
Professor and Chair, Department of Surgery
Evanston Northwestern Healthcare
Evanston, Illinois

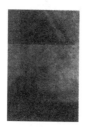

AJCC
CANCER STAGING
ATLAS

AMERICAN JOINT COMMITTEE ON CANCER
Executive Office
633 North Saint Clair Street
Chicago, Illinois 60611

FOUNDING ORGANIZATIONS
American Cancer Society
American College of Physicians
American College of Radiology
American College of Surgeons
College of American Pathologists
National Cancer Institute

SPONSORING ORGANIZATIONS
American Cancer Society
American College of Surgeons
American Society of Clinical Oncology
Centers for Disease Control and Prevention

LIAISON ORGANIZATIONS
American Urological Association
Association of American Cancer Institutes
National Cancer Registrars Association
North American Association of Central Cancer Registries
American Society of Colon and Rectal Surgeons
Society of Gynecologic Oncologists
Society of Urologic Oncology

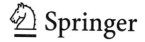 Springer

American Joint Committee on Cancer
Executive Office
633 North Saint Clair Street
Chicago, IL 60611, USA

Editors:

Frederick L. Greene, M.D.   Carolyn C. Compton, M.D., PH.D.
April G. Fritz, C.T.R., R.H.I.T.   Jatin P. Shan, M.D.
David P. Winchester, M.D.

Illustrator: Alice Y. Chen

This atlas was prepared and published through the support of the American Cancer Society, the American College of Surgeons, the American Society of Clinical Oncology, the Centers for Disease Control and Prevention, and the International Union Against Cancer.

Library of Congress Control Number: 2005932559

ISBN-10: 0-387-29014-1
ISBN-13: 978-0387-29014-0

Printed on acid-free paper.

Printed in the United States of America.   (BS/EB)

9 8 7 6 5 4 3 2 1

springeronline.com

Preface

This first edition of the *AJCC Cancer Staging Atlas* has been created as a compendium to the *AJCC Cancer Staging Manual* and *Handbook* which have now been developed through six editions and which continue to promulgate the importance of anatomical and pathological staging in the management of cancer. This *Atlas* has been viewed as a companion to illustrate the TNM classifications of all the regions included under the head and neck, digestive, thoracic, musculoskeletal, soft tissue, breast, genital, urinary and gynecologic sites. This monograph has been fully illustrated to give meaningful visualization to the TNM classifications and stage groupings and will serve as a useful reference for the clinician and patient alike.

Since there have been changes in staging strategies in the 6th Edition of the *AJCC Cancer Staging Manual*, the differences between the 5th edition and 6th edition have been included throughout the *Atlas*. This will provide a meaningful comparison for the experienced clinician as well as serve as a teaching reference for the student and trainee.

The 432 outstanding illustrations have been developed exclusively for the *AJCC Cancer Staging Atlas* by Alice Y. Chen, our exceptional medical illustrator. Every illustration provides detailed and thorough anatomic depictions to clarify critical structures and to allow the reader to instantly visualize the progressive extent of malignant disease. Appropriate labeling has been incorporated to identify significant anatomic structures. A significant number (28%) of the illustrations are devoted solely to the representation of the TNM changes which are new in the *AJCC Cancer Staging Manual*, 6th Edition. Throughout all anatomic sites, the newly developed illustrations reflect concepts that are more completely discussed in the *AJCC Cancer Staging Manual* and *Handbook*.

The *AJCC Cancer Staging Atlas* is an official publication of the American Joint Committee on Cancer and reinforces the AJCC's position as the leader in disseminating state of the art information on TNM staging. The AJCC continues to have as its mission the education of physicians, registrars and patients. The *Atlas*, a portable and easily referenced representation of the AJCC monographs, continues to enhance this mission. This project has been fully supported by our publishing colleagues at Springer and especially Laura diZerega and Bill Curtis, our longtime friends and AJCC supporters.

The editors of this most recent AJCC project wish to reinforce the concept that TNM is a universal "language" which must be applied by all clinicians caring for the cancer patients. In order to make this language come alive, a pictorial representation of clinical and pathological staging is necessary. We dedicate this work to all of our patients and colleagues and hope that they too will benefit from this illustrated resource.

Frederick L. Greene, M.D.
Carolyn C. Compton, M.D., PH.D.
April G. Fritz, C.T.R., R.H.I.T.
Jatin P. Shah, M.D.
David P. Winchester, M.D.

Contents

Purpose and Principles of Staging

PHILOSOPHY OF CLASSIFICATION AND STAGING BY THE TNM SYSTEM

A clinically useful classification scheme for cancer must encompass the attributes of the tumor that define its behavior. The American Joint Committee on Cancer (AJCC) classification is based on the premise that cancers of the same anatomic site and histology share similar patterns of growth and similar outcomes.

As the size of the untreated primary cancer (T) increases, regional lymph node involvement (N) and/or distant metastasis (M) become more frequent. A simple classification scheme, which can be incorporated into a form for staging and can be universally applied, is the goal of the TNM system as proposed by the AJCC. This classification is identical to that of the *International Union Against Cancer* (UICC).

The three significant events in the life history of a cancer—local tumor growth (T), spread to regional lymph nodes (N), and metastasis (M)—are used as they appear (or do not appear) on clinical examination, before definitive therapy begins, to indicate the anatomic extent of the cancer. This shorthand method of indicating the extent of disease (TNM) at a particular designated time is an expression of the stage of the cancer at that time in its progression.

Spread to regional lymph nodes and/or distant metastasis occur before they are discernible by clinical examination. Thus, examination during the surgical procedure and histologic examination of the surgically removed tissues may identify significant additional indicators of the prognosis of the patient (T, N, and M) as different from what could be discerned clinically before therapy. Because this is the pathologic (pTNM) classification and stage grouping (based on examination of a surgically resected specimen with sufficient tissue to evaluate the highest T, N, or M classification), it is recorded in addition to the clinical classification. It does not replace the clinical classification. Both should be maintained in the patient's permanent medical record. The clinical stage is used as a guide to the selection of primary therapy. The pathologic stage can be used as a guide to the need for adjuvant therapy, to estimation of prognosis, and to reporting end results.

Therapeutic procedures, even if not curative, may alter the course and life history of a cancer patient. Although cancers that recur after therapy may be staged with the same criteria that are used in pretreatment clinical staging, the significance of these criteria may not be the same. Hence, the "restage" classification of recurrent cancer (rTNM) is considered separately for therapeutic guidance, estimation of prognosis, and end-results reporting at that time in the patient's clinical course.

The significance of the criteria for defining anatomic extent of disease differs for tumors at different anatomic sites and of different histologic types. Therefore, the criteria for T, N, and M must be defined for tumors of each anatomic site to attain validity. With certain types of tumors, such as Hodgkin's disease and lymphomas, a different system for designating the extent of the disease and its prognosis, and for classifying its stage grouping, is necessary to achieve validity. In these exceptional circumstances, other symbols or descriptive criteria are used in place of T, N, and M.

The combination of the T, N, and M classifications into stage groupings is thus a method of designating the anatomic extent of a cancer and is related to the natural history of the particular type of cancer. It is intended to provide a means by which this information can readily be communicated to others, to assist in therapeutic decisions, and to help estimate prognosis. Ultimately, it provides a mechanism for comparing similar groups of patients when evaluating different potential therapies.

For most cancer sites, the staging recommendations in this atlas are concerned only with the anatomic extent of disease, but in several instances, histologic grade (soft-tissue sarcoma) and age (thyroid carcinoma) are factors that significantly influence prognosis and must be considered. In the future, biologic markers or genetic mutations may have to be included along with those of anatomic extent in classifying cancer, but at present they are supplements to, and not necessarily components of, the TNM stage based on anatomic extent of the cancer.

In addition to anatomic extent, the histologic type and histologic grade of the tumor may be important prognostic determinants in the classification for staging. These factors are also important variables affecting choices of treatment. For sarcomas, the tumor grade may prove to be the most important variable.

Philosophy of Changes. The introduction of new types of therapeutic interventions or new technologies may require modification of the classification and staging systems. These dynamic processes may alter treatment and outcomes. It is essential to recognize the kinetics of change of staging systems. However, changes in the staging system make it difficult to compare outcomes of current therapy with those of past treatment. Because of this, changes to the staging system must be undertaken with caution. In this edition, only factors validated in multiple large studies have been incorporated into the staging system.

NOMENCLATURE OF THE MORPHOLOGY OF CANCER

Cancer therapy decisions are made after an assessment of the patient and the tumor, using many methods that often include sophisticated technical procedures. For most types of cancer, the anatomic extent to which the disease has spread is probably the most important factor determining prognosis and must be given prime consideration in evaluating and comparing different therapeutic regimens.

Staging classifications are based on documentation of the anatomic extent of disease, and their design requires a thorough knowledge of the natural history of each type of cancer. Such knowledge has been and continues to be derived primarily from morphologic studies, which also provide us with the definitions and classifications of tumor types.

An accurate histologic diagnosis, therefore, is an essential element in a meaningful evaluation of the tumor. In certain types of cancer, biochemical, molecular, genetic, or immunologic measurements of normal or abnormal cellular function have become important elements in classifying tumors precisely. Increasingly, definitions and classifications should include function as a component of the pathologist's anatomic diagnosis. One may also anticipate that special techniques such as immunohistochemistry, cytogenetics, and molecular markers will be used more routinely for characterizing tumors and their behavior.

The most comprehensive and best-known English-language compendium of the macroscopic and microscopic characteristics of tumors and their associated behavior is the *Atlas of Tumor Pathology* series, published in many volumes by the Armed Forces Institute of Pathology in Washington, DC. These are revised periodically and are used as a basic reference by pathologists throughout the world.

RELATED CLASSIFICATIONS

Since 1958 the World Health Organization (WHO) has had a program aimed at providing internationally acceptable criteria for the histologic classification of tumors of various anatomic sites. This has resulted in the *International Histological Classification of Tumours*, which contains, in an illustrated 25-volume series, definitions, descriptions, and multiple illustrations of tumor types and proposed nomenclature.

The *WHO International Classification of Diseases for Oncology* (ICD-O). Third Edition, is a numerical coding system for neoplasms by topography and morphology. The coded morphology nomenclature is identical to the morphology field for neoplasms in the *Systematized Nomenclature of Medicine* (SNOMED) published by the College of American Pathologists.

In the interest of promoting national and international collaboration in cancer research, and specifically to facilitate appropriate comparison of data among different clinical investigations, use of the *International Histological Classification of Tumours* for classification and definition of tumor types, and use of the ICD-O codes for storage and retrieval of data, are recommended.

BIBLIOGRAPHY

Atlas of tumor pathology, 3rd series. Washington, DC: Armed Forces Institute of Pathology, 1991–2002.

International Union Against Cancer (UICC): prognostic factors in cancer, 2nd ed. Gospodarowicz MK, Henson DE, Hutter RVP, O'Sullivan B, Sobin LH, Wittekind Ch (Eds.). New York: Wiley-Liss, 2001.

International Union Against Cancer (UICC) TNM supplement: a commentary on uniform use, 2nd ed. Wittekind Ch, Henson DE, Hutter RVP, Sobin LH (Eds.). New York: Wiley-Liss, 2001.

World Health Organization: ICD-O International classification of diseases for oncology, 3rd ed. Geneva: WHO, 2000.

World Health Organization: International histological classification of tumours, 2nd ed. Berlin-Heidelberg. New York: Springer-Verlag, 1988–1997.

GENERAL RULES FOR STAGING OF CANCER

The practice of dividing cancer cases into groups according to stage arose from the observation that survival rates were higher for cases in which the disease was localized than for those in which the disease had extended beyond the organ or site of origin. These groups were often referred to as "early cases" and "late cases," implying some regular progression with time. Actually, the stage of disease at the time of diagnosis may be a reflection not only of the rate of growth and extension of the neoplasm, but also of the type of tumor and of the tumor-host relationship.

The staging of cancer is used to analyze and compare groups of patients. It is preferable to reach agreement on the recording of accurate information about the anatomic extent of the disease for each site, because the precise clinical description and histopathologic classification of malignant neoplasms may serve a number of related objectives, such as (1) selection of primary and adjuvant therapy, (2) estimation of prognosis, (3) assistance in evaluation of the results of treatment, (4) facilitation of the exchange of information among treatment centers, and (5) contribution to the continuing investigation of human cancers.

The principal purpose served by international agreement on the classification of cancer cases by anatomic extent of disease, however, is to provide a method of conveying clinical experience to others without ambiguity.

There are many classification schemes: the clinical and pathologic anatomic extent of disease; the reported duration of symptoms or signs; the sex and age of the patient; and the histologic type and grade. All of these represent variables that are known to affect or can predict the outcome of the patient. Classification by anatomic extent of disease as determined clinically and histopathologically (when possible) is the classification to which the attention of the AJCC and the UICC is primarily directed.

The clinician's immediate task is to select the most effective course of treatment and estimate the prognosis. This decision and this judgment require, among other things, an objective assessment of the anatomic extent of the disease.

To meet these stated objectives, a system of classification is needed that (1) has basic principles applicable to all anatomic sites regardless of treatment, and (2) allows the clinical appraisal to be supplemented by later information derived from surgery, histopathology, and other staging studies. The TNM system fulfills these requirements.

GENERAL RULES OF THE TNM SYSTEM

The TNM system is an expression of the anatomic extent of disease and is based on the assessment of three components:

T   The extent of the primary tumor
N   The absence or presence and extent of regional lymph node metastasis
M   The absence or presence of distant metastasis

The use of numerical subsets of the TNM components indicates the progressive extent of the malignant disease.

T0, T1, T2, T3, T4
N0, N1, N2, N3
M0, M1

In effect, the system is a shorthand notation for describing the clinical and pathologic anatomic extent of a particular malignant tumor. The following general rules apply to all sites.

1. All cases should use the following time guidelines for evaluating stage: through the first course of surgery or 4 months, whichever is longer.
2. All cases should be confirmed microscopically for TNM classification (including clinical classification). Rare cases that do not have biopsy or cytology of the tumor can be staged but should be analyzed separately and should not be included in survival analyses.
3. Four classifications are described for each site:
   - *Clinical classification*, designated **cTNM** or **TNM**
   - *Pathologic classification*, designated **pTNM**
   - *Retreatment classification*, designated **rTNM**
   - *Autopsy classification*, designated **aTNM**

Clinical classification is based on evidence acquired before primary treatment. Clinical assessment uses information available prior to first definitive treatment, including but not limited to physical examination, imaging, endoscopy, biopsy, and surgical exploration. Clinical stage is assigned prior to any cancer-directed treatment and is not changed on the basis of subsequent information. Clinical staging ends if a decision is made not to treat the patient. The clinical stage is essential to selecting and evaluating primary therapy.

Pathologic classification uses the evidence acquired before treatment, supplemented or modified by the additional evidence acquired during and from surgery, particularly from pathologic examination. The pathologic stage provides additional precise data used for estimating prognosis and calculating end results.

- The pathologic assessment of the primary tumor (pT) entails resection of the primary tumor sufficient to evaluate the highest pT category and, with several partial removals, may necessitate an effort at reasonable reconstruction to approximate the native size prior to manipulation.
- The complete pathologic assessment of the regional lymph nodes (pN) ideally entails removal of a sufficient number of lymph nodes to evaluate the highest pN category.

Exception: Sentinel node assessment may be appropriate for some sites and is clarified in chapter guidelines for those sites.*

*Note: The sentinel lymph node is the first lymph node to receive lymphatic drainage from a primary tumor. If it contains metastatic tumor, this indicates that other lymph nodes may contain tumor. If it does not contain metastatic tumor, other lymph nodes are not likely to contain tumor. Occasionally there is more than one sentinel lymph node.

- If pathologic assessment of lymph nodes reveals negative nodes but the number of examined lymph nodes is less than the suggested number for lymph node dissection, classify the N category as pN0.
- Isolated tumor cells (ITC) are single tumor cells or small clusters of cells not more than 0.2 mm in greatest dimension that are usually detected by immunohistochemistry or molecular methods. Cases with ITC in lymph nodes or at distant sites should be classified as N0 or M0, respectively. The same applies to cases with findings suggestive of tumor cells or their components by nonmorphologic techniques such as flow cytometry or DNA analysis. These cases should be analyzed separately and have special recording rules in the specific organ site.

- The pathologic assessment of metastases may be either clinical or pathologic when the T and/or N categories meet the criteria for pathologic staging (pT, pN, cM, or pM).

Pathologic classification of the extent of the primary tumor (T) and lymph nodes (N) is essential. Pathologic staging depends on the proven anatomic extent of disease, whether or not the primary lesion has been completely removed. If a biopsied primary tumor technically cannot be removed, or when it is unreasonable to remove it, and if the highest T and N categories or the M1 category of the tumor can be confirmed microscopically, the criteria for pathologic classification and staging have been satisfied without total removal of the primary cancer.

Retreatment classification is assigned when further treatment (such as chemotherapy) is planned for a caner that recurs after a disease-free interval. All information available at the time of retreatment should be used in determining the stage of the recurrent tumor (**rTNM**). Biopsy confirmation of the recurrent cancer is useful if clinically feasible, but with pathologic proof of the primary site, clinical evidence of distant metastases (usually by radiographic or related methodologies) may be used.

Autopsy classification occurs when classification of a cancer by postmortem examination is done after the death of a patient (cancer was not evident prior to death). The classification of the stage is identified as **aTNM** and includes all pathologic information obtained at the time of death.

4. **Stage grouping.** After the assignment of cT, cN, and cM and/or pT, pN, and pM categories, these may be grouped into stages. Both TNM classifications and stage groupings, once established, remain in the medical record. If there is doubt concerning the T, N, or M classification to which a particular case should be assigned, then the lower (less advanced) category should be assigned. The same principle applies to the stage grouping. Carcinoma *in situ* (CIS) is an exception to the stage grouping guidelines. By definition, CIS has not involved any structures in the primary organ that would allow tumor cells to spread to regional nodes or distant sites. Therefore, pTis, cN0, cM0, clinical stage group 0 is appropriate.

5. **Multiple tumors.** In the case of multiple, simultaneous tumors in one organ, the tumor with the highest T category is the one selected for classification and staging, and the multiplicity or the number of tumors is indicated in parentheses: for example, T2(m) or T2(5). For simultaneous bilateral cancers in paired organs, the tumors are classified separately as independent tumors in different organs. In the case of tumors of the thyroid, liver, and ovary, multiplicity is a criterion of T classification.

6. **Subsets of TNM.** Definitions of TNM categories and stage grouping may be telescoped (expanded as subsets of existing classifications) for research purposes as long as the original definitions are not changed. For instance, any of the published T, N, or M classifications can be divided into subgroups for testing and, if validated, may be submitted to the American Joint Committee on Cancer or the TNM Process Subcommittee of the UICC to be evaluated for inclusion in the classification system.

7. **Unknown primary.** In the case of a primary of unknown origin, staging can only be based on clinical suspicion of the primary origin (e.g., T0 N1 M0).

ANATOMIC REGIONS AND SITES

The sites in this classification are listed by code number of the *International Classification of Diseases for Oncology*, Third Edition (ICD-O Third Edition, World Health Organization, 2000).

DEFINITIONS OF TNM

Primary Tumor (T)

TX	Primary tumor cannot be assessed
T0	No evidence of primary tumor
Tis	Carcinoma *in situ*
T1, T2, T3 T4	Increasing size and/or local extent of the primary tumor

Regional Lymph Nodes (N)

NX	Regional lymph nodes cannot be assessed
N0	No regional lymph node metastasis
N1, N2, N3	Increasing involvement of regional lymph nodes

Note: Direct extension of the primary tumor into a lymph node(s) is classified as a lymph node metastasis.

Note: Metastasis in any lymph node other than regional is classified as a distant metastasis.

Distant Metastasis (M)

MX	Distant metastasis cannot be assessed
M0	No distant metastasis
M1	Distant metastasis

Note: For pathologic stage grouping, if sufficient tissue to evaluate the highest T and N categories has been removed for pathologic examination, M1 may be either clinical (cM1) or pathologic (pM1). If only a metastasis has had microscopic confirmation, the classification is pathologic (pM1) and the stage is pathologic.

The category M1 may be further specified according to the following notation:

Pulmonary	PUL
Osseous	OSS
Hepatic	HEP
Brain	BRA
Lymph nodes	LYM
Bone marrow	MAR
Pleura	PLE
Peritoneum	PER
Adrenals	ADR
Skin	SKI
Other	OTH

Subdivisions of TNM. Subdivisions of some main categories are available for those who need greater specificity (e.g., T1a, 1b or N2a, 2b as with breast and prostate).

HISTOLOGIC GRADE (G)

The histologic grade is a qualitative assessment of the differentiation of the tumor expressed as the extent to which a tumor resembles the normal tissue at that site. Grade is expressed in numerical grades of differentiation from most differentiated (Grade 1) to least differentiated (Grade 4), e.g., squamous cell carcinoma, moderately differentiated, Grade 2. The term *grade* is also used when other predictive, tissue-based parameters are used for prediction, particularly nuclear grade and mitotic count.

GX   Grade cannot be assessed
G1   Well differentiated
G2   Moderately differentiated
G3   Poorly differentiated
G4   Undifferentiated

For the purpose of this atlas, Grade has been included only in those chapters in which it appears in the Stage Grouping: bone, soft tissue sarcoma, and prostate.

DESCRIPTORS

For identification of special cases of TNM or pTNM classifications, the m suffix and "y," "r," and "a" prefixes are used. Although they do not affect the stage grouping, they indicate cases that require separate analysis.

m Suffix. Indicates the presence of multiple primary tumors in a single site and is recorded in parentheses: pT(m)NM.

y Prefix. Indicates those cases in which classification is performed during or following initial multimodality therapy. The cTNM or pTNM category is identified by a "y" prefix. The ycTNM or ypTNM categorizes the extent of tumor actually present at the time of that examination. The "y" categorization is not an estimate of the extent of tumor prior to multimodality therapy.

r Prefix. Indicates a recurrent tumor when staged after a disease-free interval, and is identified by the "r" prefix: rTNM. (See reclassification, r above as rTNM).

a Prefix. Designates the stage determined at autopsy: aTNM.

OTHER DESCRIPTORS

Lymphatic Vessel Invasion (L)
LX   Lymphatic vessel invasion cannot be assessed
L0   No lymphatic vessel invasion
L1   Lymphatic vessel invasion

Venous Invasion (V)
VX   Venous invasion cannot be assessed
V0   No venous invasion
V1   Microscopic venous invasion
V2   Macroscopic venous invasion

Residual Tumor (R)

The absence or presence of residual tumor after treatment is described by the symbol R.

TNM and pTNM describe the anatomic extent of cancer in general without consideration of treatment. TNM and pTNM can be supplemented by the R classification, which deals with the tumor status after treatment. It reflects the effects of therapy, influences further therapeutic procedures, and is a strong predictor of prognosis.

The R categories are

RX Presence of residual tumor cannot be assessed
R0 No residual tumor
R1 Microscopic residual tumor
R2 Macroscopic residual tumor

STAGE GROUPING

Classification by the TNM system achieves reasonably precise description and recording of the anatomic extent of disease. A tumor with 4 categories of T, 3 categories of N, and 2 categories of M has 24 TNM combinations. For purposes of tabulation and analysis, except in very large series, it is necessary to condense these combinations into a convenient number of TNM stage groupings.

The grouping adopted ensures, as far as possible, that each stage group is relatively homogencous with respect to survival and that the survival rates of these stage groupings for each cancer site are distinct. Carcinoma *in situ* is categorized Stage 0; for most sites, a case with distant metastasis is categorized Stage IV. Stages I, II, and III indicated relatively greater anatomic extent of cancer within the range from Stage 0 to Stage IV.

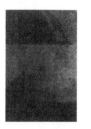

PART I
Head and Neck Sites

Introduction to Head and Neck Sites

SUMMARY OF CHANGES

- Across the board for all head and neck sites, a uniform description of advanced tumors has been recommended whereby T4 lesions are divided into T4a (resectable) and T4b (unresectable). This will allow assignment of patients with advanced stage disease to three categories: Stage IVA, advanced resectable disease; Stage IVB, advanced unresectable disease; and Stage IVC, advanced distant metastatic disease.

- In general, every effort has been made to bring the stage groupings to a relatively uniform combination of T, N, and M categories for all sites, including paranasal sinuses, salivary tumors, and thyroid tumors.

- No changes have been made in the N staging for any sites except that a descriptor has been added for nodal metastasis in the upper neck or in the lower neck, designated by (U) and (L) respectively. This descriptor will not influence nodal staging.

INTRODUCTION

Cancers of the head and neck may arise from any of the lining membranes of the upper aerodigestive tract. The T classifications indicating the extent of the primary tumor are generally similar but differ in specific details for each site because of anatomic considerations. The N classification for cervical lymph node metastasis is uniform for all mucosal sites except nasopharynx. The N classifications for thyroid and nasopharynx are unique to those sites and are based on tumor behavior and prognosis. The staging systems presented in this section are all clinical staging based on the best estimate of the extent of disease before first treatment. Imaging techniques (computed tomography [CT], magnetic resonance imaging [MRI], and ultrasonography) may be applied and, in more advanced tumor stages, have added to the accuracy of primary (T) and nodal (N) staging, especially in the nasopharyngeal, paranasal sinuses, and regional lymph nodal areas. Appropriate imaging studies should be obtained whenever the clinical findings are uncertain. Similarly, endoscopic evaluation of the primary tumor, when appropriate, is desirable for detailed assessment of the primary tumor for accurate T staging. Fine-needle aspiration (FNAB) may confirm the presence of tumor and its histopathologic nature, but it cannot rule out the presence of tumor.

Any diagnostic information that contributes to the overall accuracy of the pretreatment assessment should be considered in clinical staging and treatment planning. When surgical treatment is carried out, cancer of the head and neck can be staged (pathologic stage [pTNM]) using all information available from clinical assessment, as well as from the pathologic study of the resected specimen. The pathologic stage does not replace the clinical stage, which should be reported as well.

In reviewing the staging systems, several changes in the T classifications as well as the stage groupings are made to reflect current practices of treatment, clinical relevance, or contemporary data. Uniform T staging for oral cavity, oropharynx, salivary, and thyroid cancers greatly simplifies the systems and will improve compliance by clinicians. T4 tumors are subdivided into advanced resectable (T4a) and advanced unresectable (T4b) categories. Regrouping of Stage IV disease for all sites into advanced resectable (Stage IVA), advanced unresectable (Stage IVB), and distant metastatic (Stage IVC) also simplifies advanced-disease staging.

Chapters 3 through 8 present the illustrated staging classification for six major head and neck regions: the oral cavity, the pharynx (nasopharynx, oropharynx, and hypopharynx), the larynx, the paranasal sinuses, the salivary glands, and the thyroid gland.

ANATOMY

Regional Lymph Nodes. The status of the regional lymph nodes in head and neck cancer is of such prognostic importance that the cervical nodes must be assessed for each patient and tumor. The lymph nodes may be subdivided into specific anatomic subsites and grouped into seven levels for ease of description.

Level I:	Submental
	Submandibular
Level II:	Upper jugular
Level III:	Mid-jugular
Level IV:	Lower jugular
Level V:	Posterior triangle (spinal accessory and transverse cervical) (upper, middle, and lower, corresponding to the levels that define upper, middle, and lower jugular nodes)
Level VI:	Prelaryngeal (Delphian)
	Pretracheal
	Paratracheal
Level VII:	Upper mediastinal
Other groups:	Sub-occipital
	Retropharyngeal
	Parapharyngeal
	Buccinator (facial)
	Preauricular
	Periparotid and intraparotid

The location of the lymph node levels conforms to the following clinical descriptions, which also correlate with surgical landmarks at the time of surgical neck exploration (Figures 2.1, 2.2, 2.3).

Level I: Contains lymph nodes in the submental and submandibular triangles bounded by the anterior and posterior bellies of the digastric muscle, and the hyoid bone inferiorly, and the body of the mandible superiorly.

Level II: Contains lymph nodes in the upper jugular lymph nodes and extends from the level of the skull base superiorly to the hyoid bone inferiorly.

Level III: Contains the middle jugular lymph nodes from the hyoid bone superiorly to the level of the lower border of the cricoid cartilage inferiorly.

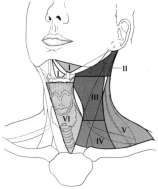

FIGURE 2.1. Schematic diagram indicating the location of the lymph node levels in the neck as described in the text.

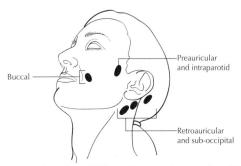

FIGURE 2.2. Location of parotid, buccal, retroauricular and occipital nodes.

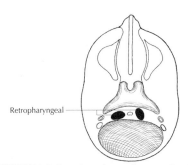

FIGURE 2.3. Location of retropharyngeal nodes.

Level IV: Contains the lower jugular lymph nodes from the level of the cricoid cartilage superiorly to the clavicle inferiorly.

Level V: Contains the lymph nodes in the posterior triangle bounded by the anterior border of the trapezius muscle posteriorly, the posterior border of the sternocleidomastoid muscle anteriorly, and the clavicle inferiorly. For descriptive purposes, Level V may be further subdivided into upper, middle, and lower levels corresponding to the superior and inferior planes that define Levels II, III, and IV.

Level VI: Contains the lymph nodes of the anterior central compartment from the hyoid bone superiorly to the suprasternal notch inferiorly. On each side, the lateral boundary is formed by the medial border of the carotid sheath.

Level VII: Contains the lymph nodes inferior to the suprasternal notch in the superior mediastinum.

The pattern of the lymphatic drainage varies for different anatomic sites. However, the location of the lymph node metastases has prognostic significance in patients with squamous cell carcinoma of the head and neck. Survival is significantly worse when metastases involve lymph nodes beyond the first echelon of lymphatic drainage and, particularly, lymph nodes in the lower region of the neck, i.e., Level IV and Level V (supraclavicular region). Consequently, it is recommended that each N staging category be recorded to show, in addition to the established parameters, whether the nodes involved are located in the upper (U) or lower (L) regions of the neck, depending on their location above or below the lower border of the cricoid cartilage.

The natural history and response to treatment of cervical nodal metastases from nasopharynx primary sites are different, in terms of their impact on prognosis, so they justify a different N classification scheme. Regional nodal metastases from well-differentiated thyroid cancer do not significantly affect the ultimate prognosis and therefore also justify a unique staging system for thyroid cancers.

Histopathologic examination is necessary to exclude the presence of tumor in lymph nodes. No imaging study (as yet) can identify microscopic tumor foci in regional nodes or distinguish between small reactive nodes and small malignant nodes.

When enlarged lymph nodes are detected, the actual size of the nodal mass(es) should be measured. It is recognized that most masses over 3 cm in diameter are not single nodes but are confluent nodes or tumor in soft tissues of the neck. Imaging studies showing amorphous spiculated margins of involved nodes or involvement of intranodal fat resulting in loss of normal oval to round nodal shape strongly suggest extracapsular (extranodal) tumor spread. Pathologic examination is necessary for documentation of tumor extent in terms of the location or level of the lymph node(s) involved, the number of nodes that contain metastases, and the presence or absence of extracapsular spread of tumor.

Metastatic Sites. The most common sites of distant spread are in the lungs and bones; hepatic and brain metastases occur less often. Mediastinal lymph node metastases are considered distant metastases.

Regional Lymph Nodes (N) (Figure 2.4)

NX   Regional lymph nodes cannot be assessed
N0   No regional lymph node metastasis
*N1   Metastasis in a single ipsilateral lymph node, 3 cm or less in greatest dimension
*N2   Metastasis in a single ipsilateral lymph node, more than 3 cm but not more than 6 cm in greatest dimension; or in multiple ipsilateral lymph nodes, none more than 6 cm in greatest dimension; or in bilateral or contralateral lymph nodes, none more than 6 cm in greatest dimension
*N2a Metastasis in single ipsilateral lymph node more than 3 cm but not more than 6 cm in greatest dimension
*N2b Metastasis in multiple ipsilateral lymph nodes, none more than 6 cm in greatest dimension
*N2c Metastasis in bilateral or contralateral lymph nodes, none more than 6 cm in greatest dimension
*N3   Metastasis in a lymph node more than 6 cm in greatest dimension

*Note: A designation of "U" or "L" may be used to indicate metastasis in the lateral neck above the lower border of the cricoid (U) or below the lower border of the cricoid (L).

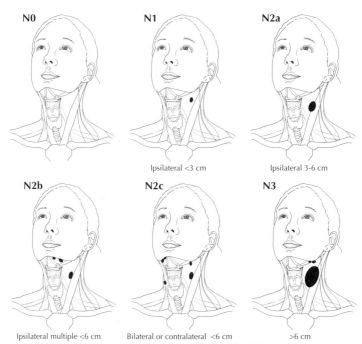

FIGURE 2.4. Regional lymph node (N) classification for all head and neck cancer sites except nasopharynx and thyroid cancers.

Distant Metastasis (M)

MX   Distant metastasis cannot be assessed

M0   No distant metastasis

M1   Distant metastasis

3

Lip and Oral Cavity

(Nonepithelial tumors such as those of lymphoid tissue, soft tissue, bone, and cartilage are not included.)

C00.0	External upper lip	C02.3	Anterior two-thirds of tongue, NOS	C04.9	Floor of mouth, NOS
C00.1	External lower lip				
C00.2	External lip, NOS	C02.8	Overlapping lesion of tongue	C05.0	Hard palate
C00.3	Mucosa of upper lip			C05.8	Overlapping lesion of palate
C00.4	Mucosa of lower lip	C02.9	Tongue, NOS		
C00.5	Mucosa of lip, NOS	C03.0	Upper gum	C05.9	Palate, NOS
C00.6	Commissure of lip	C03.1	Lower gum	C06.0	Cheek mucosa
C00.8	Overlapping lesion of lip	C03.9	Gum, NOS	C06.1	Vestibule of mouth
		C04.0	Anterior floor of the mouth	C06.2	Retromolar area
C00.9	Lip, NOS			C06.8	Overlapping lesion of other and unspecified parts of mouth
C02.0	Dorsal surface of tongue, NOS	C04.1	Lateral floor of the mouth		
C02.1	Border of tongue	C04.8	Overlapping lesion of floor of mouth	C06.9	Mouth, NOS
C02.2	Ventral surface of tongue, NOS				

SUMMARY OF CHANGES

• T4 lesions have been divided into T4a (resectable) and T4b (unresectable), leading to the division of Stage IV into Stage IVA, Stage IVB, and Stage IVC.

ANATOMY

Primary Site. The oral cavity extends from the skin-vermillion junction of the lips to the junction of the hard and soft palate above and to the line of circumvallate papillae below (Figures 3.1, 3.2, 3.3, 3.4) and is divided into the following specific:

Sites Lip. The lip begins at the junction of the vermillion border with the skin and includes only the vermillion surface or that portion of the lip that comes into contact with the opposing lip. It is well defined into an upper and lower lip joined at the commissures of the mouth.

Buccal Mucosa. This includes all the membrane lining of the inner surface of the cheeks and lips from the line of contact of the opposing lips to the line of attachment of mucosa to the alveolar ridge (upper and lower) and pterygomandibular raphe.

Lower Alveolar Ridge. This refers to the mucosa overlying the alveolar process of the mandible which extends from the line of attachment of mucosa in the buccal gutter to the line of free mucosa of the floor of the mouth. Posteriorly it extends to the ascending ramus of the mandible.

Upper Alveolar Ridge. This refers to the mucosa overlying the alveolar process of the maxilla which extends from the line of attachment of mucosa in the upper

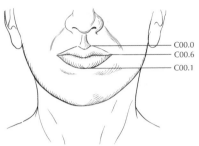

FIGURE 3.1. Anatomical subsites of the lip.

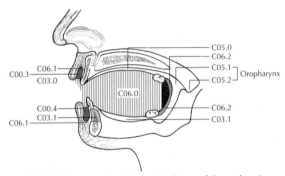

FIGURE 3.2. Anatomical sites and subsites of the oral cavity.

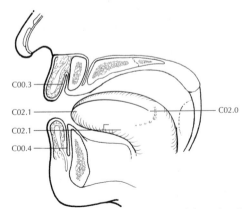

FIGURE 3.3. Anatomical sites and subsites of the oral cavity.

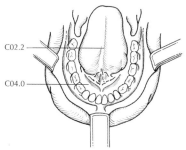

FIGURE 3.4. Anatomical sites and subsites of the oral cavity.

gingival buccal gutter to the junction of the hard palate. Its posterior margin is the upper end of the pterygopalatine arch.

Retromolar Gingiva (Retromolar Trigone). This is the attached mucosa overlying the ascending ramus of the mandible from the level of the posterior surface of the last molar tooth to the apex superiorly, adjacent to the tuberosity of the maxilla.

Floor of the Mouth. This is a semilunar space over the myelohyoid and hyoglossus muscles, extending from the inner surface of the lower alveolar ridge to the undersurface of the tongue. Its posterior boundary is the base of anterior pillar of the tonsil. It is divided into two sides by the frenulum of the tongue and contains the ostia of the submaxillary and sublingual salivary glands.

Hard Palate. This is the semilunar area between the upper alveolar ridge and mucous membrane covering the palatine process of the maxillary palatine bones. It extends from the inner surface of the superior alveolar ridge to the posterior edge of the palatine bone.

Anterior Two-thirds of the Tongue (Oral Tongue). This is the freely mobile portion of the tongue that extends anteriorly from the line of circumvallate papillae to the undersurface of the tongue at the junction of the floor of the mouth. It is composed of four areas: the tip, the lateral borders, the dorsum, and the undersurface (nonvillous ventral surface of the tongue). The undersurface of the tongue is considered a separate category by the World Health Organization (WHO).

Regional Lymph Nodes. Mucosal cancer of the oral cavity may spread to regional lymph node(s). Tumors of each anatomic site have their own predictable patterns of regional spread. The risk of regional metastases is generally related to the T category and, probably more important, to the depth of infiltration of the primary tumor. Cancer of the lip carries a low metastatic risk and initially involves adjacent submental and submandibular nodes, then jugular nodes. Cancers of the hard palate and alveolar ridge likewise have a low metastatic potential and involve buccinator, submandibular, jugular, and occasionally retropharyngeal nodes. Other oral cancers will spread primarily to submandibular and jugular nodes and uncommonly to posterior triangle/supraclavicular nodes. Cancer of the anterior oral tongue may spread directly to lower jugular nodes. The closer to the midline the primary, the greater the risk of bilateral cervical nodal spread. Any previous treatment to the neck, surgical and/or radiation, may alter normal lymphatic drainage patterns, resulting in unusual distribution of regional spread of disease to the cervical lymph nodes. In general, cervical lymph node involvement from oral cavity primary sites is predictable and orderly, spreading from the primary to upper, then middle, and subsequently lower cervical nodes. However, disease in the anterior oral cavity may also spread directly to the mid-cervical lymph nodes. The risk of distant metastasis is more dependent on the N than on the T status of the head and neck cancer. Midline nodes are considered ipsilateral. In addition to the components to describe the N category, regional lymph nodes should also be described according to the level of the neck that is involved. It is recognized that the level of involved nodes in the neck is prognostically significant (lower is worse), as is the presence of extracapsular extension of metastatic tumor from individual nodes. Imaging studies showing amorphous spiculated margins of involved nodes or involvement of internodal fat resulting in loss of normal oval-to-round nodal shape strongly suggest extracapsular (extranodal) tumor spread; however, pathologic examination is necessary for documentation of the extent of such disease. No imaging study (as yet) can identify microscopic foci of cancer in regional nodes or distinguish between small reactive nodes and small malignant nodes (unless central radiographic inhomogeneity is present). For pN, a selective neck dissection will ordinarily include six or more lymph nodes, and a radical or modified radical neck dissection will ordinarily include 10 or more lymph nodes. Negative pathologic examination of a lesser number of nodes still mandates a pN0 designation.

Metastatic Sites. The lungs are the commonest site of distant metastases; skeletal and hepatic metastases occur less often. Mediastinal lymph node metastases are considered distant metastases.

DEFINITIONS

Primary Tumor (T)

TX   Primary tumor cannot be assessed
T0   No evidence of primary tumor
Tis Carcinoma *in situ*
T1   Tumor 2 cm or less in greatest dimension (Figures 3.5A, B)
T2   Tumor more than 2 cm but not more than 4 cm in greatest dimension (Figures 3.6A, B)
T3   Tumor more than 4 cm in greatest dimension (Figures 3.7A–C)
T4a (Lip) Tumor invades through cortical bone, inferior alveolar nerve, floor of mouth, or skin of face, i.e., chin or nose[1] (Figure 3.8)
T4a (Oral Cavity) Tumor invades through cortical bone, into deep [extrinsic] muscle of tongue (genioglossus, hyoglossus, palatoglossus, and styloglossus), maxillary sinus, or skin of face (Figure 3.9)
T4b Tumor involves masticator space, pterygoid plates, or skull base and/or encases internal carotid artery (Figure 3.10)

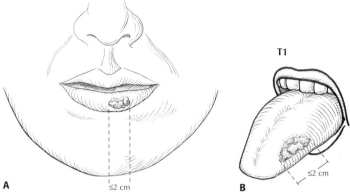

FIGURE 3.5. A. T1 is defined as a tumor 2 cm or less in greatest dimension. **B.** T1 is defined as a tumor 2 cm or less in greatest dimension.

Regional Lymph Nodes (N) (see Figure 2.4)

NX Regional lymph nodes cannot be assessed
N0 No regional lymph node metastasis
N1 Metastasis in a single ipsilateral lymph node, 3 cm or less in greatest dimension
N2 Metastasis in a single ipsilateral lymph node, more than 3 cm but not more than 6 cm in greatest dimension; or in multiple ipsilateral lymph nodes, none more than 6 cm in greatest dimension; or in bilateral or contralateral lymph nodes, none more than 6 cm in greatest dimension

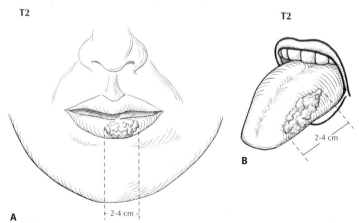

FIGURE 3.6. A. T2 is defined as a tumor more than 2 cm but not more than 4 cm in greatest dimension. **B.** T2 is defined as a tumor more than 2 cm but not more than 4 cm in greatest dimension.

T3

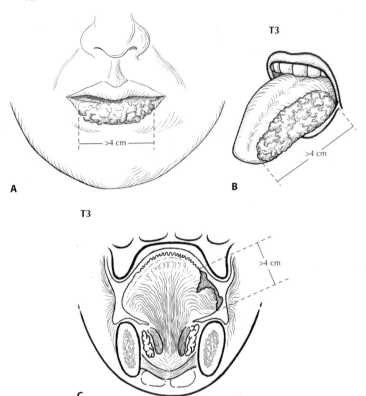

FIGURE 3.7. A. T3 is defined as tumor more than 4 cm in greatest dimension. **B.** T3 is defined as tumor more than 4 cm in greatest dimension. **C.** T3 is defined as tumor more than 4 cm in greatest dimension.

T4 (Lip)

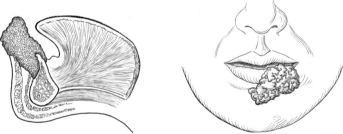

FIGURE 3.8. T4a (Lip) is defined as tumor invading through cortical bone, inferior alveolar nerve, floor of mouth, or skin of face, i.e., chin or nose (as shown).[1]

T4a (Oral Cavity)

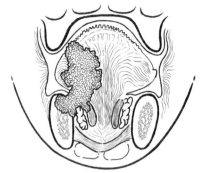

FIGURE 3.9. T4a (Oral Cavity) is defined as tumor invading through cortical bone, into deep [extrinsic] muscle of tongue (genioglossus, hyoglossus, palatoglossus, and styloglossus), maxillary sinus, or skin of face.

N2a   Metastasis in single ipsilateral lymph node more than 3 cm but not more than 6 cm in greatest dimension

N2b   Metastasis in multiple ipsilateral lymph nodes, none more than 6 cm in greatest dimension

N2c   Metastasis in bilateral or contralateral lymph nodes, none more than 6 cm in greatest dimension

N3   Metastasis in a lymph node more than 6 cm in greatest dimension

Distant Metastasis (M)

MX   Distant metastasis cannot be assessed

M0   No distant metastasis

M1   Distant metastasis

T4b

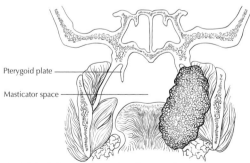

Pterygoid plate

Masticator space

FIGURE 3.10. T4b is defined as tumor involves masticator space, pterygoid plates (as shown), or skull base and/or encases internal carotid artery.

STAGE GROUPING

0	Tis	N0	M0
I	T1	N0	M0
II	T2	N0	M0
III	T3	N0	M0
	T1	N1	M0
	T2	N1	M0
	T3	N1	M0
IVA	T4a	N0	M0
	T4a	N1	M0
	T1	N2	M0
	T2	N2	M0
	T3	N2	M0
	T4a	N2	M0
IVB	Any T	N3	M0
	T4b	Any N	M0
IVC	Any T	Any N	M1

NOTE

1. Superficial erosion alone of bone/tooth socket by gingival primary is not sufficient to classify as T4.

Pharynx (Including Base of Tongue, Soft Palate, and Uvula)

(Nonepithelial tumors, such as those of lymphoid tissue, soft tissue, bone, and cartilage, are not included.)

C01.9	Base of tongue, NOS	C10.4	Branchial cleft	C13.0	Postcricoid region
		C10.8	Overlapping lesion	C13.1	Hypopharyngeal
C02.4	Lingual tonsil	C10.9	Oropharynx, NOS		aspect of aryepiglottic
C05.1	Soft palate, NOS	C11.0	Superior wall of		fold
C05.2	Uvula		nasopharynx	C13.2	Posterior wall of
C09.0	Tonsillar fossa	C11.1	Posterior wall of		hypopharnyx
C09.1	Tonsillar pillar		nasopharynx	C13.8	Overlapping lesion
C09.8	Overlapping lesion	C11.2	Lateral wall of	C13.9	Hypopharnyx,
C09.9	Tonsil, NOS		nasopharynx		NOS
C10.0	Vallecula	C11.3	Anterior wall of	C14.0	Pharynx, NOS
C10.2	Lateral wall of		nasopharynx	C14.2	Waldeyer's ring
	oropharynx	C11.8	Overlapping lesion	C14.8	Overlapping lesion of
C10.3	Posterior pharyngeal	C11.9	Nasopharynx, NOS		lip, oral cavity, and
	wall	C12.9	Pyriform sinus		pharynx

> **SUMMARY OF CHANGES**
>
> • For oropharynx and hypopharynx only, T4 lesions have been divided into T4a (resectable) and T4b (unresectable), leading to the division of Stage IV into Stage IVA, Stage IVB, and Stage IVC.

ANATOMY

Primary Sites and Subsites. The pharynx is divided into three regions: nasopharynx, oropharynx, and hypopharynx (Figures 4.1, 4.2, 4.3). Each region is further subdivided into specific sites as summarized in the following:

Nasopharynx. The nasopharynx begins anteriorly at the posterior choana and extends along the plane of the airway to the level of the free border of the soft palate. It includes the vault, the lateral walls (including the fossae of Rosenmuller and the mucosa covering the torus tubaris forming the Eustachian tube orifice), and the posterior wall. The floor is the superior surface of the soft palate. The posterior margins of the choanal orifices and of the nasal septum are included in the nasal fossa.

Parapharyngeal involvement denotes posterolateral infiltration of tumor beyond the pharyngobasilar fascia. Involvement of the masticator space denotes extension of tumor beyond the anterior surface of the lateral pterygoid muscle, or lateral extension beyond the posterolateral wall of the maxillary antrum, and the pterygomaxillary fissure.

Oropharynx. The oropharynx is the region in continuity of the pharynx extending from the plane of the superior surface of the soft palate to the superior surface of the hyoid bone (or floor of the vallecula). It includes the base of the

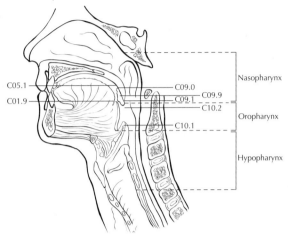

FIGURE 4.1. Sagittal view of the face and neck depicting the subdivisions of the pharynx as described in the text.

tongue, the inferior (anterior) surface of the soft palate and the uvula, the anterior and posterior tonsillar pillars, the glossotonsillar sulci, the pharyngeal tonsils, and the lateral and posterior pharyngeal walls.

Hypopharynx. The hypopharynx is that portion of the pharynx extending from the plane of the superior border of the hyoid bone (or floor of the vallecula) to the plane corresponding to the lower border of the cricoid cartilage. It connects

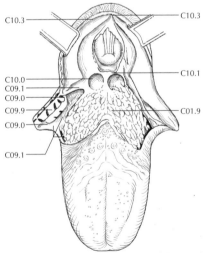

FIGURE 4.2. Anatomical sites and subsites of the oropharynx.

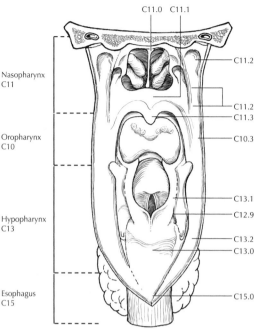

FIGURE 4.3. Anatomical sites and subsites of the nasopharynx, oropharynx, hypopharynx, and esophagus.

the two pyriform sinuses at the post cricoid region, thus forming the anterior wall of the hypopharynx. The pyriform sinus extends from the pharyngoepiglottic fold to the upper end of the esophagus at the lower border of the cricoid cartilages. The posterior pharyngeal wall extends from the level of the superior surface of the hyoid bone (or floor of the vallecula) to the inferior border of the cricoid cartilage and from the apex of one pyriform sinus to the other.

Regional Lymph Nodes. The risk of regional lymph nodal spread from cancers of the pharynx is high. Primary nasopharyngeal tumors commonly spread to retropharyngeal, upper jugular, and spinal accessory nodes, often bilaterally. Oropharyngeal cancers involve upper and mid-jugular lymph nodes and (less commonly) submental/submandibular nodes. Hypopharyngeal cancers spread to adjacent parapharyngeal, paratracheal, and mid- and lower jugular nodes. Bilateral lymphatic drainage is common.

In clinical evaluation, the maximum size of the nodal mass should be measured. Most masses over 3 cm in diameter are not single nodes but, rather, are confluent nodes or tumor in soft tissues of the neck. There are three categories of clinically involved nodes for the nasopharynx, oropharynx, and hypopharynx: N1, N2, and N3. The use of subgroups a, b, and c is not required but is recommended. Midline nodes are considered ipsilateral nodes. In addition to the components to describe the N category, regional lymph nodes should also be described according to the level of the neck that is involved. The level of involved nodes in the neck is prognostically significant (lower is worse), as is the presence of extracapsular extension of metastatic tumor from individual nodes. Imaging studies showing amorphous spiculated margins of involved nodes or involvement of internodal fat resulting in loss of normal oval-to-round nodal shape strongly suggest extracapsular (extranodal) tumor spread; however, pathologic examination is necessary for documentation of such disease extent. No imaging study (as yet) can identify microscopic foci of cancer in regional nodes or distinguish between small reactive nodes and small malignant nodes (unless central radiographic inhomogeneity is present). For pN, a selective neck dissection will ordinarily include six or more lymph nodes, and a radical or modified radical neck dissection will ordinarily include 10 or more lymph nodes. Negative pathologic examination of a lesser number of nodes still mandates a pN0 designation.

Metastatic Sites. The lungs are the commonest site of distant metastases; skeletal and hepatic metastases occur less often. Mediastinal lymph node metastases are considered distant metastases.

DEFINITIONS

Primary Tumor (T)
TX   Primary tumor cannot be assessed
T0   No evidence of primary tumor
Tis   Carcinoma *in situ*

Nasopharynx
T1   Tumor confined to the nasopharynx (Figure 4.4)
T2   Tumor extends to soft tissues (Figure 4.4)
T2a   Tumor extends to the oropharynx and/or nasal cavity without parapharyngeal extension[1] (Figure 4.5)
T2b   Any tumor with parapharyngeal extension[1] (Figure 4.6)
T3   Tumor involves bony structures and/or paranasal sinuses (Figure 4.7)

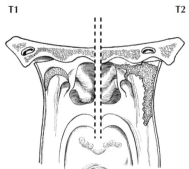

FIGURE 4.4. For nasopharynx, T1 is defined as tumor confined to the nasopharynx (left) whereas T2 extends to soft tissues.

T2a

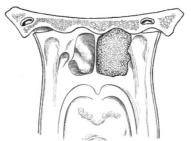

FIGURE 4.5. T2a is defined as tumor extending to the oropharynx and/or nasal cavity without parapharyngeal extension.

T2b

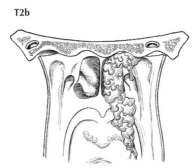

FIGURE 4.6. T2b is defined as any nasopharynx tumor with parapharyngeal extension.

T3

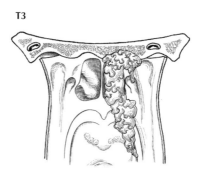

FIGURE 4.7. T3 tumors involve bony structures and/or paranasal sinuses.

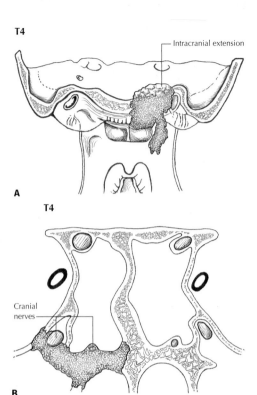

T4

Intracranial extension

A

T4

Cranial nerves

B

FIGURE 4.8. A,B. T4 is defined as a tumor with intracranial extension (A) and/or involvement of cranial nerves (B), infratemporal fossa, hypopharynx, orbit, or masticator space.

T4   Tumor with intracranial extension and/or involvement of cranial nerves, infratemporal fossa, hypopharynx, orbit, or masticator space (Figures 4.8A, B)

Oropharynx

T1   Tumor 2 cm or less in greatest dimension (Figure 4.9)

T2   Tumor more than 2 cm but not more than 4 cm in greatest dimension (Figure 4.10)

T3   Tumor more than 4 cm in greatest dimension (Figure 4.11)

T4a   Tumor invades the larynx, deep/extrinsic muscle of tongue, medial pterygoid, hard palate, or mandible (Figure 4.12)

T4b   Tumor invades lateral pterygoid muscle, pterygoid plates, lateral nasopharynx, or skull base or encases carotid artery (Figure 4.13)

Hypopharynx

T1   Tumor limited to one subsite of hypopharynx and 2 cm or less in greatest dimension (Figures 4.14A–C)

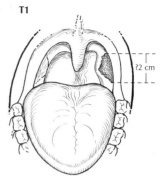

FIGURE 4.9. T1 tumors of the oropharynx are 2 cm or less in greatest dimension and are confined to one subsite.

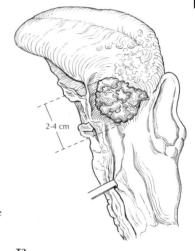

FIGURE 4.10. T2 tumors of the oropharynx invade more than one subsite or an adjacent site and measure more than 2 cm but not more than 4 cm.

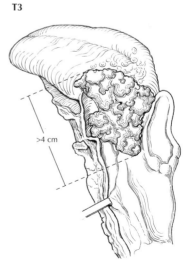

FIGURE 4.11. T3 tumors of the oropharynx are more than 4 cm in greatest dimension.

T4a

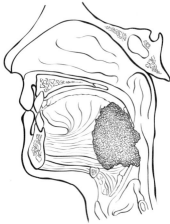

FIGURE 4.12. T4a tumor of the oropharynx is described as a tumor that invades the larynx, deep/extrinsic music of tongue, medial pterygoid, hard plate, or mandible.

T2 Tumor invades more than one subsite of hypopharynx or an adjacent site, or measures more than 2 cm but not more than 4 cm in greatest diameter without fixation of hemilarynx (Figures 4.15A–E)

T3 Tumor measures more than 4 cm in greatest dimension or with fixation of hemilarynx (Figures 4.16A–C)

T4b

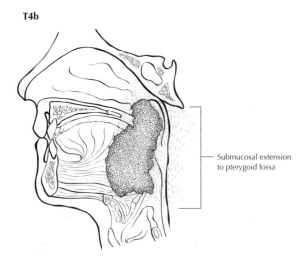

— Submucosal extension to pterygoid fossa

FIGURE 4.13. T4b tumor of oropharynx showing submucosal extension to the pterygoid fossa.

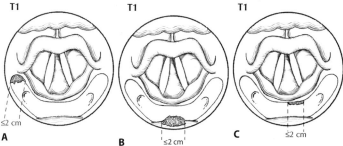

FIGURE 4.14. A. T1 tumor of the hypopharynx with involvement of the pyriform sinus. **B.** T1 tumor of the hypopharynx with involvement of the posterior wall. **C.** T1 tumor of the hypopharynx with involvement of the post-cricoid area.

4

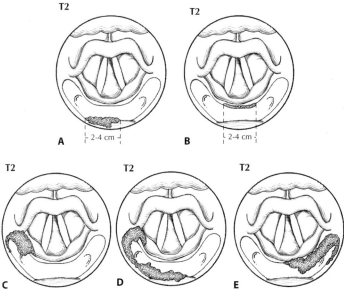

FIGURE 4.15. A. T2 tumor of the hypopharynx with involvement of the posterior wall of the hypopharynx. **B.** T2 tumor of the hypopharynx with involvement of the post-cricoid area. **C.** T2 tumor of the hypopharynx with involvement of the pyriform sinus and the aryepiglottic fold. **D.** T2 tumor of the hypopharynx with involvement of the pyriform sinus and the posterior wall. **E.** T2 tumor of the hypopharynx with involvement of the pyriform sinus and the post-cricoid area.

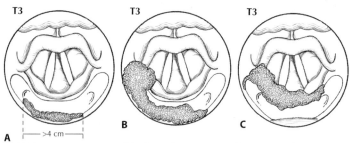

FIGURE 4.16. A. T3 tumor of the hypopharynx greater than 4 cm in diameter and with involvement of the posterior wall. **B.** T3 tumor of the hypopharynx with fixation of the hemilarynx and invasion of the pyriform sinus, aryepiglottic fold, and posterior wall. **C.** T3 tumor of the hypopharynx with fixation of the hemilarynx with invasion of the pyriform sinus and post-cricoid area.

T4a Tumor invades thyroid/cricoid cartilage, hyoid bone, thyroid gland, esophagus or central compartment soft tissue[2] (Figures 4.17A, B)

T4b Tumor invades prevertebral fascia, encases carotid artery, or involves mediastinal structures (Figure 4.18)

Regional Lymph Nodes (N)

Nasopharynx
The distribution and the prognostic impact of regional lymph node spread from nasopharynx cancer (particularly of the undifferentiated type) are different from those of other head and neck mucosal cancers and justify the use of a different N classification scheme as illustrated in Figures 4.19, 4.20, and 4.21.

NX Regional lymph nodes cannot be assessed
N0 No regional lymph node metastasis

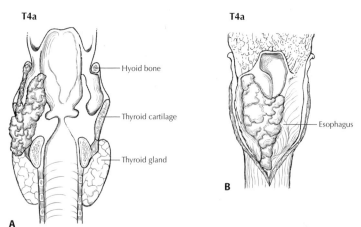

FIGURE 4.17. A. T4a tumor of the hypopharynx with invasion of the hyoid bone, thyroid cartilage and thyroid gland. **B.** T4a tumor of the hypopharynx with invasion of the esophagus.

T4b

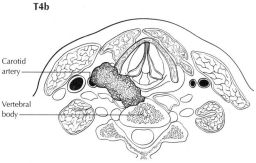

FIGURE 4.18. T4b tumor the hypopharynx with invasion of the carotid artery and prevertebral fascia.

4

N1

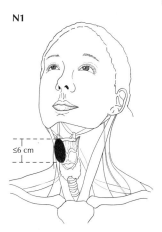

FIGURE 4.19. N1 for nasopharynx cancer is defined as unilateral metastasis in lymph node(s), 6 cm or less in greatest dimension, above the supraclavicular fossa.

N2

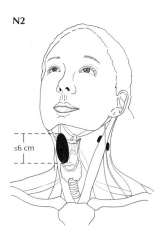

FIGURE 4.20. N2 for nasopharynx cancer is defined as bilateral metastasis in lymph node(s), 6 cm or less in greatest dimension, above the supraclavicular fossa.

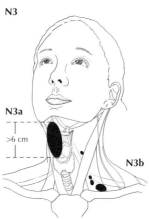

FIGURE 4.21. N3 for nasopharynx cancer may be categorized as N3a (left) for metastasis in a lymph node(s) greater than 6 cm in dimension and/or N3b (right) metastatic to the supraclavicular fossa.

N1   Unilateral metastasis in lymph node(s), 6 cm or less in greatest dimension, above the supraclavicular fossa[3] (Figure 4.19)

N2   Bilateral metastasis in lymph node(s), 6 cm or less in greatest dimension, above the supraclavicular fossa[3] (Figure 4.20)

N3   Metastasis in a lymph node(s) >6 cm and/or to supraclavicular fossa

N3a   Greater than 6 cm in dimension (Figure 4.21)

N3b   Extension to the supraclavicular fossa[3] (Figure 4.21)

Oropharynx and Hypopharynx (see Figure 2.4)

NX   Regional lymph nodes cannot be assessed

N0   No regional lymph node metastasis

N1   Metastasis in a single ipsilateral lymph node, 3 cm or less in greatest dimension

N2   Metastasis in a single ipsilateral lymph node, more than 3 cm but not more than 6 cm in greatest dimension, or in multiple ipsilateral lymph nodes, none more than 6 cm in greatest dimension, or in bilateral or contralateral lymph nodes, none more than 6 cm in greatest dimension

N2a   Metastasis in a single ipsilateral lymph node more than 3 cm but not more than 6 cm in greatest dimension

N2b   Metastasis in multiple ipsilateral lymph nodes, none more than 6 cm in greatest dimension

N2c   Metastasis in bilateral or contralateral lymph nodes, none more than 6 cm in greatest dimension

N3   Metastasis in a lymph node more than 6 cm in greatest dimension

Distant Metastasis (M)

MX   Distant metastasis cannot be assessed

M0   No distant metastasis

M1   Distant metastasis

STAGE GROUPING: NASOPHARYNX

0	Tis	N0	M0
I	T1	N0	M0
IIA	T2a	N0	M0
IIB	T1	N1	M0
	T2	N1	M0
	T2a	N1	M0
	T2b	N0	M0
	T2b	N1	M0
III	T1	N2	M0
	T2a	N2	M0
	T2b	N2	M0
	T3	N0	M0
	T3	N1	M0
	T3	N2	M0
IVA	T4	N0	M0
	T4	N1	M0
	T4	N2	M0
IVB	Any T	N3	M0
IVC	Any T	Any N	M1

STAGE GROUPING: OROPHARYNX AND HYPOPHARYNX

0	Tis	N0	M0
I	T1	N0	M0
II	T2	N0	M0
III	T3	N0	M0
	T1	N1	M0
	T2	N1	M0
	T3	N1	M0
IVA	T4a	N0	M0
	T4a	N1	M0
	T1	N2	M0
	T2	N2	M0
	T3	N2	M0
	T4a	N2	M0
IVB	T4b	Any N	M0
	Any T	N3	M0
IVC	Any T	Any N	M1

NOTES

1. Parapharyngeal extension denotes posterolateral infiltration of tumor beyond the pharyngobasilar fascia.
2. Central compartment soft tissue includes prelaryngeal strap muscles and subcutaneous fat.
3. Midline nodes are considered ipsilateral nodes.

Larynx

(Nonepithelial tumors such as those of lymphoid tissue, soft tissue, bone, and cartilage are not included.)

C10.1	Anterior (lingual) surface of epiglottis	C32.1	Supraglottis (laryngeal surface)	C32.8	Overlapping lesion of larynx
C32.0	Glottis	C32.2	Subglottis	C32.9	Larynx, NOS
		C32.2	Laryngeal cartilage		

SUMMARY OF CHANGES

- T4 lesions have been divided into T4a (resectable) and T4b (unresectable), leading to the division of Stage IV into Stage IVA, Stage IVB, and Stage IVC.

ANATOMY

Primary Site. The following anatomic definition of the larynx allows classification of carcinomas arising in the encompassed mucous membranes but excludes cancers arising on the lateral or posterior pharyngeal wall, pyriform fossa, postcricoid area, or base of tongue.

The anterior limit of the larynx is composed of the anterior or lingual surface of the suprahyoid epiglottis, the thyrohyoid membrane, the anterior commissure, and the anterior wall of the subglottic region, which is composed of the thyroid cartilage, the cricothyroid membrane, and the anterior arch of the cricoid cartilage.

The posterior and lateral limits include the laryngeal aspect of the aryepiglottic folds, the arytenoid region, the interarytenoid space, and the posterior surface of the subglottic space, represented by the mucous membrane covering the surface of the cricoid cartilage.

The superolateral limits are composed of the tip and the lateral borders of the epiglottis. The inferior limits are made up of the plane passing through the inferior edge of the cricoid cartilage.

For purposes of this clinical stage classification, the larynx is divided into three regions: supraglottis, glottis, and subglottis (Figures 5.1, 5.2). The supraglottis is composed of the epiglottis (both its lingual and laryngeal aspects), aryepiglottic folds (laryngeal aspects), arytenoids, and the ventricular bands (false cords). The epiglottis is divided for staging purposes into suprahyoid and infrahyoid portions by a plane at the level of the hyoid bone. The inferior boundary of the supraglottis is a horizontal plane passing through the lateral margin of the ventricle at its junction with the superior surface of the vocal cord. The glottis is composed of the superior and inferior surfaces of the true vocal cords, including the anterior and posterior commissures. It occupies a horizontal plane 1 cm in thickness, extending inferiorly from the lateral margin of the ventricle. The subglottis is the region extending from the lower boundary of the glottis to the lower margin of the cricoid cartilage.

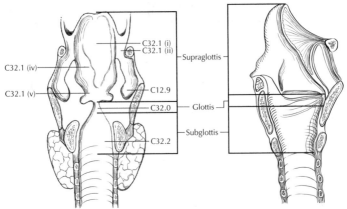

FIGURE 5.1. Anatomical sites and subsites of the three regions of the larynx: supraglottis, glottis, and subglottis. Supraglottis (C32.1) subsites include suprahyoid epiglottis (i), aryepiglottic fold, laryngeal aspect (ii), infrahyoid epiglottis (iv), and ventricular bands or false cords (v).

The division of the larynx is summarized as follows:

Site	*Subsite*
Supraglottis	Suprahyoid epiglottis
	Infrahyoid epiglottis
	Aryepiglottic folds (laryngeal aspect)
	Arytenoids
	Ventricular bands (false cords)
Glottis	True vocal cords, including anterior and posterior commissures
Subglottis	Subglottis

Regional Lymph Nodes. The incidence and distribution of cervical nodal metastases from cancer of the larynx vary with the site of origin and the T classification of the primary tumor. The true vocal cords are nearly devoid of lymphatics, and tumors of that site alone rarely spread to regional nodes. By

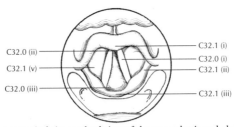

FIGURE 5.2. Anatomical sites and subsites of the supraglottis and glottis. Supraglottis (C32.1) subsites include suprahyoid epiglottis (i), aryepiglottic fold, laryngeal aspect (ii), arytenoids (iii), and ventricular bands or false cords (v). Glottis (C32.0) subsites include vocal cords (i), anterior commissure (ii), and posterior commissure (iii).

contrast, the supraglottis has a rich and bilaterally interconnected lymphatic network, and primary supraglottic cancers are commonly accompanied by regional lymph node spread. Glottic tumors may spread directly to adjacent soft tissues and prelaryngeal, pretracheal, paralaryngeal, and paratracheal nodes, as well as to upper, mid-, and lower jugular nodes. Supraglottic tumors commonly spread to upper and midjugular nodes, considerably less commonly to submental or submandibular nodes, and occasionally to retropharyngeal nodes. The rare subglottic primary tumors spread first to adjacent soft tissues and prelaryngeal, pretracheal, paralaryngeal and paratracheal nodes, then to mid- and lower jugular nodes. Contralateral lymphatic spread is common.

In clinical evaluation, the physical size of the nodal mass should be measured. Most masses over 3 cm in diameter are not single nodes but, rather, are confluent nodes or tumor in soft tissues of the neck. There are three categories of clinically positive nodes: N1, N2, and N3. Midline nodes are considered ipsilateral nodes. In addition to the components to describe the N category, regional lymph nodes should also be described according to the level of the neck that is involved. Pathologic examination is necessary for documentation of such disease extent. Imaging studies showing amorphous spiculated margins of involved nodes or involvement of internodal fat resulting in loss of normal oval-to-round nodal shape strongly suggest extracapsular (extranodal) tumor spread; however, pathologic examination is necessary for documentation of such disease extent. No imaging study (as yet) can identify microscopic foci of cancer in regional nodes or distinguish between small reactive nodes and small malignant nodes without central radiographic inhomogeneity.

Metastatic Sites. Distant spread is common only for patients who have bulky regional lymphadenopathy. When distant metastases occur, spread to the lungs is most common; skeletal or hepatic metastases occur less often. Mediastinal lymph node metastases are considered distant metastases.

DEFINITIONS

Primary Tumor (T)

TX Primary tumor cannot be assessed
T0 No evidence of primary tumor
Tis Carcinoma *in situ*

Supraglottis
T1 Tumor limited to one subsite of supraglottis with normal vocal cord mobility (Figures 5.3A, B)
T2 Tumor invades mucosa of more than one adjacent subsite of supraglottis or glottis or region outside the supraglottis (e.g., mucosa of base of tongue, vallecula, medial wall of pyriform sinus) without fixation of the larynx (Figures 5.4A, B)
T3 Tumor limited to larynx with vocal cord fixation and/or invades any of the following: postcricoid area, pre-epiglottic tissues, paraglottic space, and/or minor thyroid cartilage erosion (e.g., inner cortex) (Figures 5.5A, B)
T4a Tumor invades through the thyroid cartilage and/or invades tissues beyond the larynx (e.g., trachea, soft tissues of neck including deep

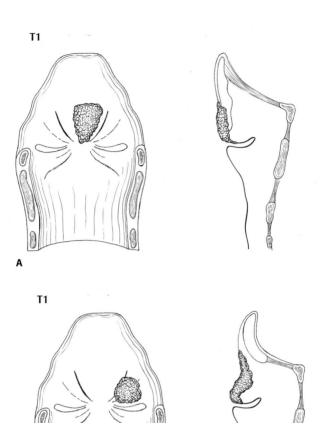

FIGURE 5.3. A. T1 is defined as tumor limited to one subsite of supraglottis (shown here in the epiglottis) with normal vocal cord mobility. **B.** T1 is defined as tumor limited to one subsite of supraglottis (shown here in the ventricular bands) with normal vocal cord mobility.

T2

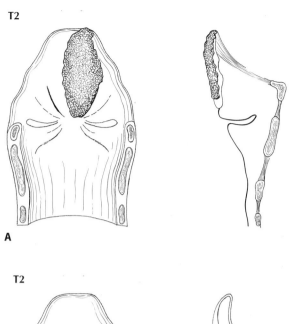

A

T2

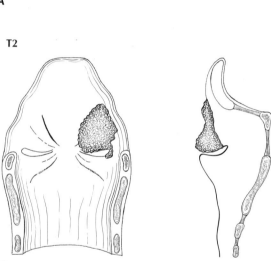

B

FIGURE 5.4. A. T2 is defined as tumor invading the mucosa of more than one adjacent subsite of supraglottis or glottis or region outside the supraglottis (e.g., mucosa of base of tongue, vallecula, medial wall of pyriform sinus) without fixation of the larynx (shown here with tumor involvement in the suprahyoid and mucosa of the infrahyoid epiglottis). **B.** T2 with invasion of ventricular bands (false cords) and the epiglottis.

T3

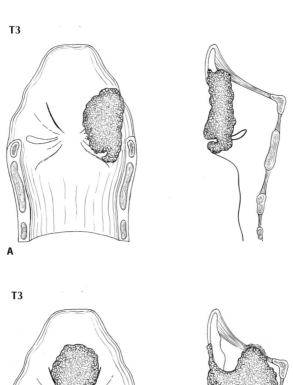

A

T3

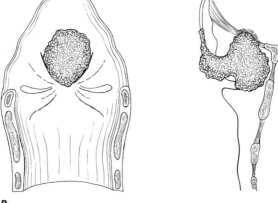

B

FIGURE 5.5. A. T3 is defined as tumor limited to larynx with vocal cord fixation and/or invading any of the following: postcricoid area, pre-epiglottic tissues, paraglottic space, and/or minor thyroid cartilage erosion (e.g., inner cortex), here with invasion of the supraglottis and vocal cord with vocal cord fixation. **B.** T3 with invasion of the pre-epiglottic tissues with vocal cord fixation.

T4a

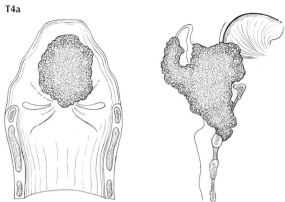

FIGURE 5.6. T4a is defined as tumor invading through the thyroid cartilage and/or invading tissues beyond the larynx (e.g., trachea, soft tissues of neck including deep extrinsic muscle of the tongue, strap muscles, thyroid, or esophagus). Here, tumor has invaded beyond the larynx into the vallecula and base of the tongue as well as into soft tissues of the neck.

extrinsic muscle of the tongue, strap muscles, thyroid, or esophagus) (Figure 5.6)

T4b   Tumor invades prevertebral space, encases carotid artery, or invades mediastinal structures (Figure 5.7)

Glottis

T1   Tumor limited to the vocal cord(s) (may involve anterior or posterior commissure) with normal mobility (Figure 5.8)

T1a Tumor limited to one vocal cord (Figure 5.8)

T1b Tumor involves both vocal cords (Figure 5.8)

T4b

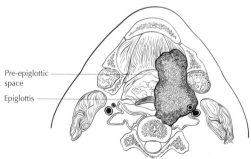

Pre-epiglottic space

Epiglottis

FIGURE 5.7. Cross-sectional illustration of T4b tumor, which is defined as invading prevertebral space, encasing the carotid artery (shown), or invading mediastinal structures.

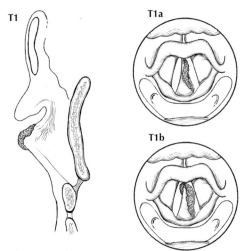

FIGURE 5.8. T1 tumors of the glottis are limited to the vocal cord(s) with normal mobility (may involve anterior or posterior commissure). T1a tumors are limited to one vocal cord (top right) and T1b tumors involve both vocal cords (bottom right).

T2　　Tumor extends to supraglottis and/or subglottis, or with impaired vocal cord mobility (Figure 5.9)

T3　　Tumor limited to the larynx with vocal cord fixation, and/or invades paraglottic space, and/or minor thyroid cartilage erosion (e.g., inner cortex) (Figure 5.10)

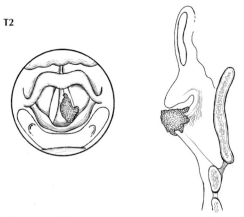

FIGURE 5.9. T2 tumors of the glottis extend to supraglottis and/or subglottis, or with impaired vocal cord mobility.

T3

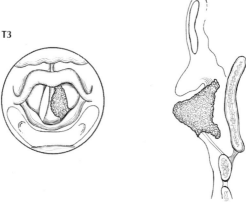

FIGURE 5.10. T3 tumors of the glottis are limited to the larynx with vocal cord fixation (shown), and/or invade paraglottic space, and/or minor thyroid cartilage erosion (e.g., inner cortex).

5

T4a Tumor invades through the thyroid cartilage and/or invades tissues beyond the larynx (e.g., trachea, soft tissues of neck including deep extrinsic muscle of the tongue, strap muscles, thyroid, or esophagus) (Figure 5.11)

T4b Tumor invades prevertebral space, encases carotid artery, or invades mediastinal structures

Subglottis

T1 Tumor limited to the subglottis (Figure 5.12)

T2 Tumor extends to vocal cord(s) with normal or impaired mobility (Figure 5.13)

T4a

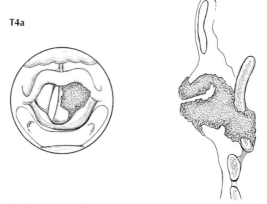

FIGURE 5.11. T4a tumors of the glottis invade through the thyroid cartilage and/or invade tissues beyond the larynx (e.g., trachea, soft tissues of neck including deep extrinsic muscle of the tongue, strap muscles, thyroid, or esophagus).

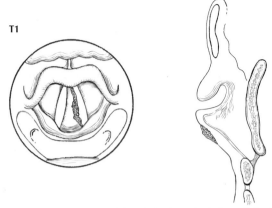

FIGURE 5.12. T1 tumors of the subglottis are limited to subglottis.

T3   Tumor limited to larynx with vocal cord fixation (Figure 5.14)

T4a   Tumor invades cricoid or thyroid cartilage and/or invades tissues beyond the larynx (e.g., trachea, soft tissues of neck including deep extrinsic muscles of the tongue, strap muscles, thyroid, or esophagus) (Figure 5.15)

T4b   Tumor invades prevertebral space, encases carotid artery, or invades mediastinal structures

Regional Lymph Nodes (N) (see Figure 2.4)

NX   Regional lymph nodes cannot be assessed

N0   No regional lymph node metastasis

N1   Metastasis in a single ipsilateral lymph node, 3 cm or less in greatest dimension

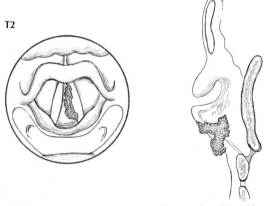

FIGURE 5.13. T2 tumors of the subglottis extend to vocal cord(s), with normal or impaired mobility.

T3

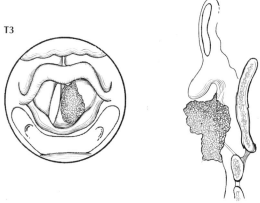

FIGURE 5.14. T3 tumors of the subglottis are limited to larynx with vocal cord fixation.

N2   Metastasis in a single ipsilateral lymph node, more than 3 cm but not more than 6 cm in greatest dimension, or in multiple ipsilateral lymph nodes, none more than 6 cm in greatest dimension, or in bilateral or contralateral lymph nodes, none more than 6 cm in greatest dimension

N2a   Metastasis in a single ipsilateral lymph node, more than 3 cm but not more than 6 cm in greatest dimension

N2b   Metastasis in multiple ipsilateral lymph nodes, none more than 6 cm in greatest dimension

N2c   Metastasis in bilateral or contralateral lymph nodes, none more than 6 cm in greatest dimension

N3   Metastasis in a lymph node, more than 6 cm in greatest dimension

T4a

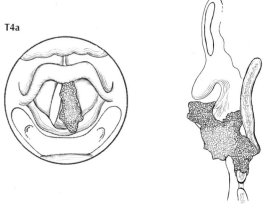

FIGURE 5.15. T4a tumors of the subglottis invade cricoid or thyroid cartilage and/or invade tissues beyond the larynx (e.g., trachea, soft tissues of neck including deep extrinsic muscles of the tongue, strap muscles, thyroid, or esophagus).

Distant Metastasis (M)

MX   Distant metastasis cannot be assessed
M0   No distant metastasis
M1   Distant metastasis

STAGE GROUPING

0	Tis	N0	M0
I	T1	N0	M0
II	T2	N0	M0
III	T3	N0	M0
	T1	N1	M0
	T2	N1	M0
	T3	N1	M0
IVA	T4a	N0	M0
	T4a	N1	M0
	T1	N2	M0
	T2	N2	M0
	T3	N2	M0
	T4a	N2	M0
IVB	T4b	Any N	M0
	Any T	N3	M0
IVC	Any T	Any N	M1

Nasal Cavity and Paranasal Sinuses

(Nonepithelial tumors such as those of lymphoid tissue, soft tissue, bone, and cartilage are not included.)

C30.0 Nasal cavity   C31.0 Maxillary sinus   C31.1 Ethmoid sinus

---

SUMMARY OF CHANGES

- A new site has been added for inclusion into the staging system. In addition to maxillary sinus, the nasoethmoid complex is described as a second site with two regions within this site: nasal cavity and ethmoid sinuses.

- The nasal cavity region is further divided into four subsites: septum, floor, lateral wall, and vestibule. The ethmoid sinus region is divided into two subsites: right and left.

- The T staging of ethmoid lesions has been revised to reflect nasoethmoid tumors, and appropriate descriptions for the T staging have been added.

- For maxillary sinus, T4 lesions have been divided into T4a (resectable) and T4b (unresectable), leading to the division of Stage IV into Stage IVA, Stage IVB, and Stage IVC.

6

ANATOMY

Primary Sites. Cancer of the maxillary sinus is the most common of the sinonasal malignancies. Ethmoid sinuses and nasal cavity cancers are equal in frequency but considerably less common than maxillary sinus cancers. Tumors of the sphenoid and frontal sinuses are rare.

The location as well as the extent of the mucosal lesion within the maxillary sinus has prognostic significance. Historically, Ohngren's line, connecting the medial canthus of the eye to the angle of the mandible, is used to divide the maxillary sinus into an anteroinferior portion (infrastructure), which is associated with a good prognosis, and a superoposterior portion (suprastructure), which has a poor prognosis (Figure 6.1). The poorer outcome associated with superoposterior cancers reflects early extension of these tumors to critical structures, including the eye, skull base, pterygoids, and infratemporal fossa.

For the purpose of staging, the nasoethmoidal complex is divided into two sites: nasal cavity and ethmoid sinuses. The ethmoids are further subdivided into two sites: left and right, separated by the nasal septum. The nasal cavity is divided into four subsites: the septum, floor, lateral wall, and vestibule.

Site	Subsite
Maxillary sinus	Left/right
Nasal cavity	Septum
	Floor
	Lateral wall
	Vestibule

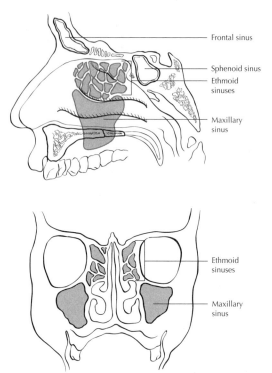

FIGURE 6.1. Sites of origin of tumors of the paranasal sinuses.

Ethmoid sinus   Left
                   Right

Regional Lymph Nodes. Regional lymph node spread from cancer of nasal cavity and paranasal sinuses is relatively uncommon. Involvement of buccinator, submandibular, upper jugular, and (occasionally) retropharyngeal nodes may occur with advanced maxillary sinus cancer which involve adjacent structures, including soft tissues of the cheek, upper alveolus, palate, and buccal mucosa. Ethmoid sinus cancers are less prone to regional lymphatic spread. When only one side of the neck is involved, it should be considered ipsilateral. Bilateral spread may occur with advanced primary cancer, particularly with spread of the primary beyond the midline.

In clinical evaluation, the physical size of the nodal mass should be measured. Most masses over 3 cm in diameter are not single nodes but, rather, are confluent nodes or tumor in soft tissues of the neck. There are three categories of clinically positive nodes: N1, N2, and N3. Midline nodes are considered ipsilateral nodes. In addition to the components to describe the N category, regional lymph nodes should also be described according to the level of the neck that is involved. Pathologic examination is necessary for documentation of such disease extent. Imaging studies showing amorphous spiculated margins of involved nodes or involvement of internodal fat resulting in loss of normal oval-to-round nodal shape strongly suggest extracapsular (extranodal) tumor spread; however, pathologic examination is necessary for documentation of such disease extent. No imaging study (as yet) can identify microscopic foci of cancer in regional nodes or distinguish between small reactive nodes and small malignant nodes without central radiographic inhomogeneity.

For pN, a selective neck dissection will ordinarily include 6 or more lymph nodes, and a radical or modified radical neck dissection will ordinarily include 10 or more lymph nodes. Negative pathologic examination of a lesser number of lymph nodes still mandates a pN0 designation.

Metastatic Disease. Distant spread usually occurs to lungs but occasionally there is spread to bone.

DEFINITIONS

Primary Tumor (T)

Maxillary Sinus

TX   Primary tumor cannot be assessed

T0   No evidence of primary tumor

Tis   Carcinoma *in situ*

T1   Tumor limited to the maxillary sinus mucosa with no erosion or destruction of bone (Figure 6.2)

T2   Tumor causing bone erosion or destruction including extension into the hard palate and/or middle nasal meatus, except extension to posterior wall of maxillary sinus and pterygoid plates (Figure 6.3)

T3   Tumor invades any of the following: bone of the posterior wall of maxillary sinus, subcutaneous tissues, floor or medial wall of orbit, pterygoid fossa, ethmoid sinuses (Figure 6.4)

T4a   Tumor invades anterior orbital contents, skin of cheek, pterygoid plates, infratemporal fossa, cribriform plate, sphenoid or frontal sinuses (Figures 6.5A, B)

T1

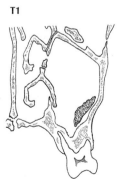

FIGURE 6.2. T1 is limited to the maxillary sinus mucosa.

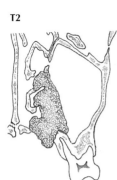

T2

FIGURE 6.3. T2 causes bone erosion or destruction including extension into the hard palate and/or middle nasal meatus with the exception of extension to posterior wall of maxillary sinus and pterygoid plates.

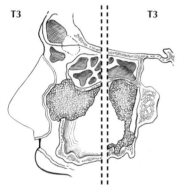

T3   **T3**   **FIGURE 6.4.** Two views of T3.

Tumor invades any of the following: bone of the posterior wall of maxillary sinus, subcutaneous tissues, floor or medial wall of orbit, pterygoid fossa, ethmoid sinuses.

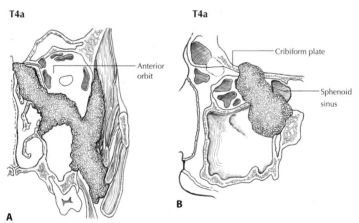

T4a   **T4a**

Anterior orbit

Cribiform plate

Sphenoid sinus

A

B

FIGURE 6.5. A. T4a showing tumor invasion of anterior orbital contents. **B.** T4a showing tumor invasion of sphenoid sinus and cribriform plate.

T4b

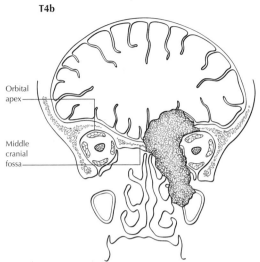

Orbital apex

Middle cranial fossa

FIGURE 6.6. Coronal view of T4b shows tumor invades orbital apex and or dura, brain or middle cranical fossa.

T4b Tumor invades any of the following: orbital apex, dura, brain, middle cranial fossa, cranial nerves other than maxillary division of trigeminal nerve V_2, nasopharynx, or clivus (Figure 6.6)

Nasal Cavity and Ethmoid Sinus

TX Primary tumor cannot be assessed
T0 No evidence of primary tumor
Tis Carcinoma *in situ*
T1 Tumor restricted to any one subsite, with or without bony invasion (Figure 6.7)

T1

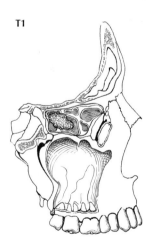

FIGURE 6.7. In the nasal cavity and ethmoid sinus, T1 is defined as tumor restricted to any one subsite, with or without bony invasion.

T2

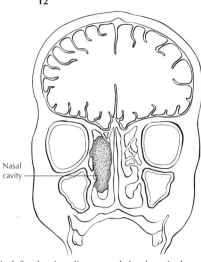

Nasal
cavity

FIGURE 6.8. T2 is defined as invading two subsites in a single region or extending to involve an adjacent region within the nasoethmoidal complex, here the nasal cavity, and ethmoid with or without bony invasion.

T2 Tumor invading two subsites in a single region or extending to involve an adjacent region within the nasoethmoidal complex, with or without bony invasion (Figure 6.8)

T3 Tumor extends to invade the medial wall or floor of the orbit, maxillary sinus, palate, or cribriform plate (Figure 6.9)

T4a Tumor invades any of the following: anterior orbital contents, skin of nose or cheek, minimal extension to anterior cranial fossa, pterygoid plates, sphenoid or frontal sinuses (Figure 6.10)

T4b Tumor invades any of the following: orbital apex, dura, brain, middle cranial fossa, cranial nerves other than V_2, nasopharynx, or clivus (Figure 6.11)

Regional Lymph Nodes (N) (see Figure 2.4)

NX Regional lymph nodes cannot be assessed

N0 No regional lymph node metastasis

N1 Metastasis in a single ipsilateral lymph node, 3 cm or less in greatest dimension

N2 Metastasis in a single ipsilateral lymph node, more than 3 cm but not more than 6 cm in greatest dimension, or in multiple ipsilateral lymph nodes, none more than 6 cm in greatest dimension, or in bilateral or contralateral lymph nodes, none more than 6 cm in greatest dimension

N2a Metastasis in a single ipsilateral lymph node, more than 3 cm but not more than 6 cm in greatest dimension

N2b Metastasis in multiple ipsilateral lymph nodes, none more than 6 cm in greatest dimension

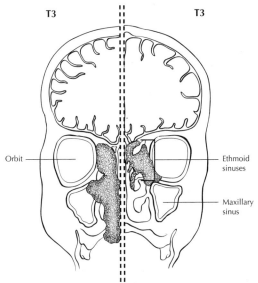

FIGURE 6.9. Two views of T3 showing tumor invading maxillary sinus and palate (left) and extending to the floor of the orbit and cribriform plate (right).

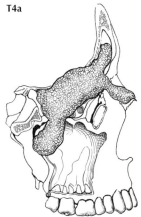

FIGURE 6.10. T4a invades any of the following: anterior orbital contents, skin of nose or cheek, minimal extension to anterior cranial fossa, pterygoid plates, sphenoid or frontal sinuses.

T4b

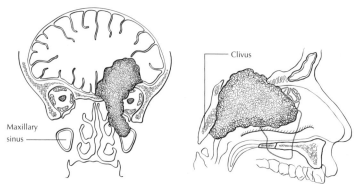

FIGURE 6.11. Two views of T4b. The coronal view on the left shows invasion in the orbital apex and brain. On the right, tumor invades the clivus.

N2c   Metastasis in bilateral or contralateral lymph nodes, none more than 6 cm in greatest dimension

N3   Metastasis in a lymph node, more than 6 cm in greatest dimension

Distant Metastasis (M)

MX   Distant metastasis cannot be assessed

M0   No distant metastasis

M1   Distant metastasis

STAGE GROUPING

0	Tis	N0	M0
I	T1	N0	M0
II	T2	N0	M0
III	T3	N0	M0
	T1	N1	M0
	T2	N1	M0
	T3	N1	M0
IVA	T4a	N0	M0
	T4a	N1	M0
	T1	N2	M0
	T2	N2	M0
	T3	N2	M0
	T4a	N2	M0
IVB	T4b	Any N	M0
	Any T	N3	M0
IVC	Any T	Any N	M1

Major Salivary Glands (Parotid, Submandibular, and Sublingual)

C07.9	Parotid gland	C08.8	Overlapping lesion of	C08.9	Major salivary gland,
C08.0	Submandibular gland		major salivary glands		NOS
C08.1	Sublingual gland				

SUMMARY OF CHANGES

- In order to maintain internal consistency of T staging across all sites, the description for T3 has been revised. In addition to tumors having extraparenchymal extension, all tumors larger than 4 cm are considered T3.

- T4 lesions have been divided into T4a (resectable) and T4b (unresectable), leading to the division of Stage IV into Stage IVA, Stage IVB, and Stage IVC.

INTRODUCTION

This staging system is based on an extensive retrospective review of the world literature regarding malignant tumors of the major salivary glands. Numerous factors affect patient survival, including the histologic diagnosis, cellular differentiation of the tumor (grade), site, size, degree of fixation or local extension, facial nerve involvement, and the status of regional lymph nodes as well as distant metastases. The classification involves the four dominant clinical variables: tumor size, local extension of the tumor, nodal metastasis, and distant metastasis. The T4 category has been divided into T4a and T4b. T4a indicates advanced lesions that are resectable with grossly clear margins; T4b reflects extension to areas that preclude resection with clear margins. Histologic grade, patient age, and tumor site are important additional factors that should be recorded for future analysis and potential inclusion in the staging system.

ANATOMY

Primary Site. The major salivary glands include the parotid, submandibular, and sublingual glands. Tumors arising in minor salivary glands (mucus-secreting glands in the lining membrane of the upper aerodigestive tract) are staged according to the anatomic site of origin (e.g., oral cavity, sinuses, etc.).

Primary tumors of the parotid constitute the largest proportion of salivary gland tumors. Sublingual primary cancers are rare and may be difficult to distinguish with certainty from minor salivary gland primary tumors of the anterior floor of the mouth.

Regional Lymph Nodes. Regional lymphatic spread from salivary gland cancer is less common than from head and neck mucosal squamous cancers and varies according to the histology and size of the primary tumor. Most nodal metastases will be clinically apparent on initial evaluation.

Low-grade tumors rarely metastasize to regional nodes, whereas the risk of regional spread is substantially higher from high-grade cancers. Regional dissemination tends to be orderly, progressing from intraglandular to adjacent (periparotid, submandibular) nodes, then to upper and midjugular nodes, and occasionally to retropharyngeal nodes. Bilateral lymphatic spread is rare.

For pN, a selective neck dissection will ordinarily include 6 or more lymph nodes, and a radical or modified radical neck dissection will ordinarily include 10 or more lymph nodes. Negative pathologic examination of a lesser number of lymph nodes still mandates a pN0 designation.

Metastatic Sites. Distant spread is most frequently to the lungs.

DEFINITIONS

Primary Tumor (T)

TX   Primary tumor cannot be assessed

T0   No evidence of primary tumor

T1   Tumor 2 cm or less in greatest dimension without extraparenchymal extension[1] (Figure 7.1)

T2   Tumor more than 2 cm but not more than 4 cm in greatest dimension without extraparenchymal extension[1] (Figure 7.2)

T3   Tumor more than 4 cm and/or tumor having extraparenchymal extension[1] (Figures 7.3A, B)

T4a   Tumor invades skin, mandible, ear canal, and/or facial nerve (Figures 7.4A–D)

T1

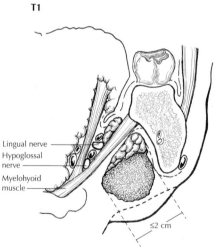

FIGURE 7.1. T1 is defined as a tumor 2 cm or less in greatest dimension without extraparenchymal extension (a coronal section thru the floor of the mouth with tumor of the submandibular gland is shown).

FIGURE 7.2. T2 is defined as a tumor greater than 2 cm but not more than 4 cm in greatest dimension without extraparenchymal extension (an axial section with tumor of the deep lobe of the parotid gland is shown).

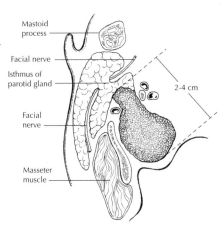

T2

Mastoid process

Facial nerve

Isthmus of parotid gland

2-4 cm

Facial nerve

Masseter muscle

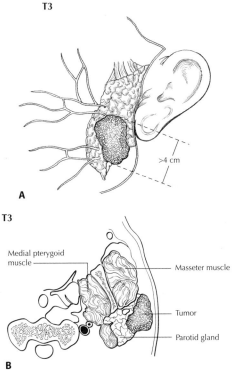

T3

>4 cm

A

T3

Medial pterygoid muscle

Masseter muscle

Tumor

Parotid gland

B

FIGURE 7.3. A. T3 is defined as greater than 4 cm and/or tumor having extraparenchymal extension (a tumor of the superficial lobe of the parotid gland is shown). **B.** Cross-sectional diagram of T3 tumor with extraparenchymal extension from the parotid gland.

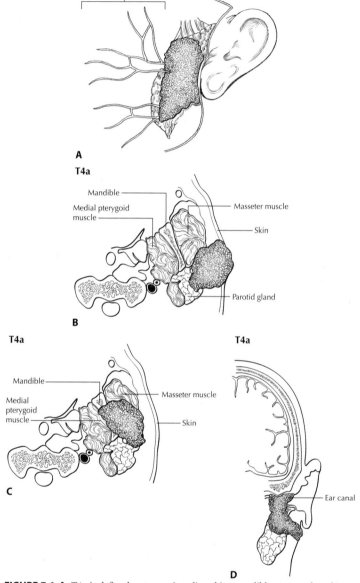

FIGURE 7.4. A. T4a is defined as tumor invading skin, mandible, ear canal, and/or facial nerve (as illustrated here). **B.** Cross-sectional diagram of T4a tumor invading skin. **C.** Cross-sectional diagram of T4a tumor invading mandible. **D.** Coronal section of T4 tumor invading ear canal.

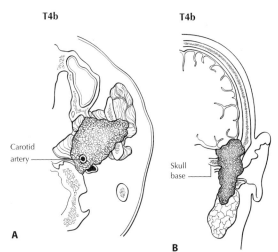

T4b   **T4b**

Carotid
artery

Skull
base

A

B

FIGURE 7.5. A. T4b is defined as tumor invading skull base and/or pterygoid plates and/or encasing carotid artery. In this cross-sectional diagram, the tumor encases the carotid artery. **B.** Coronal section of T4b tumor invading skull base.

T4b   Tumor invades skull base and/or pterygoid plates and/or encases carotid artery (Figures 7.5A, B)

Regional Lymph Nodes (N) (see Figure 2.4)

NX   Regional lymph nodes cannot be assessed
N0   No regional lymph node metastasis
N1   Metastasis in a single ipsilateral lymph node, 3 cm or less in greatest dimension
N2   Metastasis in a single ipsilateral lymph node, more than 3 cm but not more than 6 cm in greatest dimension, or in multiple ipsilateral lymph nodes, none more than 6 cm in greatest dimension, or in bilateral or contralateral lymph nodes, none more than 6 cm in greatest dimension
N2a   Metastasis in a single ipsilateral lymph node, more than 3 cm but not more than 6 cm in greatest dimension
N2b   Metastasis in multiple ipsilateral lymph nodes, none more than 6 cm in greatest dimension
N2c   Metastasis in bilateral or contralateral lymph nodes, none more than 6 cm in greatest dimension
N3   Metastasis in a lymph node, more than 6 cm in greatest dimension

Distant Metastasis (M)

MX   Distant metastasis cannot be assessed
M0   No distant metastasis
M1   Distant metastasis

STAGE GROUPING

I	T1	N0	M0
II	T2	N0	M0
III	T3	N0	M0
	T1	N1	M0
	T2	N1	M0
	T3	N1	M0
IVA	T4a	N0	M0
	T4a	N1	M0
	T1	N2	M0
	T2	N2	M0
	T3	N2	M0
	T4a	N2	M0
IVB	T4b	Any N	M0
	Any T	N3	M0
IVC	Any T	Any N	M1

NOTE

1. Extraparenchymal extension is clinical or macroscopic evidence of invasion of soft tissues. Microscopic evidence alone does not constitute extraparenchymal extension for classification purposes.

Thyroid

C73.9   Thyroid gland

SUMMARY OF CHANGES

- Tumor staging (T) has been revised and the categories redefined.

- T4 is now divided into T4a and T4b.

- Nodal staging (N) has been revised.

- All anaplastic carcinomas are considered T4. The T4 category for anaplastic carcinomas is divided into T4a (intrathyroidal anaplastic carcinoma—surgically resectable) and T4b (extrathyroidal anaplastic carcinoma—surgically unresectable).

- For papillary and follicular carcinomas, the stage grouping for patients older than 45 has been revised. Stage III includes tumors with minimal extrathyroid extension. Stage IVA includes tumors of any size extending beyond the thyroid capsule to invade subcutaneous soft tissues, larynx, trachea, esophagus, or recurrent laryngeal nerve. Stage IVB includes tumors that invade prevertebral fascia, carotid artery, or mediastinal vessels. Stage IVC includes advanced tumors with distant metastasis.

INTRODUCTION

Although staging for cancers in other head and neck sites is based entirely on the anatomic extent of disease, it is not possible to follow this pattern for the unique group of malignant tumors that arise in the thyroid gland. Both the *histologic diagnosis* and the *age* of the patient are of such importance in the behavior and the prognosis of thyroid cancer that these factors are included in this staging system.

ANATOMY

Primary Site. The thyroid gland ordinarily is composed of a right and a left lobe lying adjacent and lateral to the upper trachea and esophagus. An isthmus connects the two lobes, and in some cases a pyramidal lobe is present extending upward anterior to the thyroid cartilage (Figure 8.1).

Regional Lymph Nodes. Regional lymph node spread from thyroid cancer is common but of less prognostic significance in patients with well-differentiated tumors (papillary, follicular) than in medullary cancers. The adverse prognostic influence of lymph node metastasis in patients with differentiated carcinomas is observed only in the older age group. The first echelon of nodal metastasis consists of paralaryngeal, paratracheal, and prelaryngeal (Delphian) nodes adjacent to the thyroid gland in the central compartment of the neck generally described as Level VI. Metastases secondarily involve the mid- and lower jugular,

---

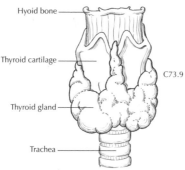

Hyoid bone

Thyroid cartilage

C73.9

Thyroid gland

Trachea

FIGURE 8.1. Thyroid gland.

the supraclavicular, and (much less commonly) the upper deep jugular and spinal accessory lymph nodes. Lymph node metastasis to submandibular and submental lymph nodes is very rare. Upper mediastinal (Level VII) nodal spread occurs frequently both anteriorly and posteriorly. Retropharyngeal nodal metastasis may be seen, usually in the presence of extensive lateral cervical metastasis. Bilateral nodal spread is common. The components of the N category are described as follows: first echelon (central compartment/Level VI) or N1a, and lateral cervical and/or superior mediastinal or N1b. The lymph node metastasis should also be described according to the level of the neck that is involved. Nodal metastases from medullary thyroid cancer carry a much more ominous prognosis, although they follow a similar pattern of spread.

For pN, histologic examination of a selective neck dissection will ordinarily include 6 or more lymph nodes, whereas histologic examination or a radical or a modified radical comprehensive neck dissection will ordinarily include 10 or more lymph nodes. Negative pathologic evaluation of a lesser number of nodes still mandates a pN0 designation.

Metastatic Sites. Distant spread occurs by hematogenous routes—for example to lungs and bones—but many other sites may be involved.

DEFINITIONS

Primary Tumor (T)
All categories may be subdivided: (a) solitary tumor, (b) multifocal tumor (the largest determines the classification).

TX   Primary tumor cannot be assessed
T0   No evidence of primary tumor
T1   Tumor 2 cm or less in greatest dimension limited to the thyroid (Figure 8.2)
T2   Tumor more than 2 cm but not more than 4 cm in greatest dimension limited to the thyroid (Figure 8.3)
T3   Tumor more than 4 cm in greatest dimension limited to the thyroid or any tumor with minimal extrathyroid extension (e.g., extension to sternothyroid muscle or perithyroid soft tissues) (Figure 8.4)

FIGURE 8.2. T1 is defined as tumor 2 cm or less in greatest dimension limited to the thyroid.

T1

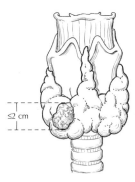

T2

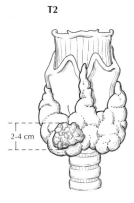

FIGURE 8.3. T2 is defined as tumor more than 2 cm but not more than 4 cm in greatest dimension limited to the thyroid.

8

T3 **T3**

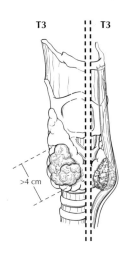

FIGURE 8.4. Two views of T3: on the left, a tumor more than 4 cm in greatest dimension limited to the thyroid; on the right, a tumor with minimal extrathyroid extension (to either sternothyroid muscle or perithyroid soft tissues).

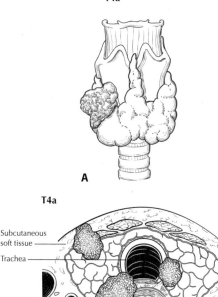

T4a

A

T4a

Subcutaneous soft tissue

Trachea

Esophagus

B

FIGURE 8.5. A. T4a is defined as a tumor of any size extending beyond the thyroid capsule to invade subcutaneous soft tissues, larynx, trachea, esophagus, or recurrent laryngeal nerve. **B.** Cross-sectional diagram of three different parameters of T4a: tumor invading subcutaneous soft tissues; tumor invading trachea; tumor invading esophagus.

T4a   Tumor of any size extending beyond the thyroid capsule to invade subcutaneous soft tissues, larynx, trachea, esophagus, or recurrent laryngeal nerve (Figures 8.5A, B)

T4b   Tumor invades prevertebral fascia or encases carotid artery or mediastinal vessels (Figure 8.6)

All anaplastic carcinomas are considered T4 tumors.

T4a   Intrathyroidal anaplastic carcinoma—surgically resectable

T4b   Extrathyroidal anaplastic carcinoma—surgically unresectable

Regional Lymph Nodes (N)
Regional lymph nodes are the central compartment, lateral cervical, and upper mediastinal lymph nodes.

NX   Regional lymph nodes cannot be assessed
N0   No regional lymph node metastasis
N1   Regional lymph node metastasis

T4b

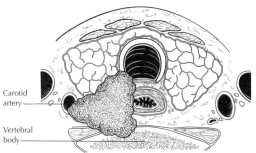

Carotid artery —

Vertebral body —

FIGURE 8.6. T4b is defined as tumor invading prevertebral fascia or encasing carotid artery or mediastinal vessels. Cross-sectional diagram of two different parameters of T4b: tumor encases carotid artery; tumor invades vertebral body.

N1a Metastasis to Level VI (pretracheal, paratracheal, and prelaryngeal/ Delphian lymph nodes) (Figure 8.7)

N1b Metastasis to unilateral, bilateral, or contralateral cervical or superior mediastinal lymph nodes (Figure 8.8)

Distant Metastasis (M)
MX Distant metastasis cannot be assessed
M0 No distant metastasis
M1 Distant metastasis

N1a

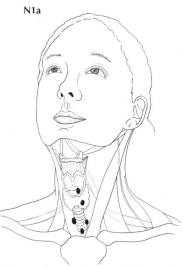

FIGURE 8.7. N1a is defined as metastasis to Level VI (pretracheal, paratracheal, and prelaryngeal/Delphian lymph nodes).

N1b

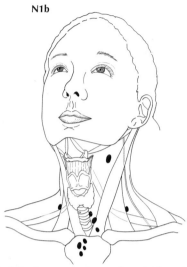

FIGURE 8.8. N1b is defined as metastasis to unilateral, bilateral, or contralateral cervical or superior mediastinal lymph nodes.

STAGE GROUPING

Separate stage groupings are recommended for papillary or follicular, medullary, and anaplastic (undifferentiated) carcinoma.

Papillary or Follicular

Under 45 years

I	Any T	Any N	M0
II	Any T	Any N	Ml

Papillary or Follicular

45 years and older

I	T1	N0	M0
II	T2	N0	M0
III	T3	N0	M0
	T1	N1a	M0
	T2	N1a	M0
	T3	N1a	M0
IVA	T4a	N0	M0
	T4a	N1a	M0
	T1	N1b	M0
	T2	N1b	M0
	T3	N1b	M0
	T4a	N1b	M0

IVB	T4b	Any N	M0
IVC	Any T	Any N	M1

Medullary Carcinoma

I	T1	N0	M0
II	T2	N0	M0
III	T3	N0	M0
	T1	N1a	M0
	T2	N1a	M0
	T3	N1a	M0
IVA	T4a	N0	M0
	T4a	N1a	M0
	T1	N1b	M0
	T2	N1b	M0
	T3	N1b	M0
	T4a	N1b	M0
IVB	T4b	Any N	M0
IVC	Any T	Any N	M1

Anaplastic Carcinoma

IVA	T4a	Any N	M0
IVB	T4b	Any N	M0
IVC	Any T	Any N	M1

8

PART II
Digestive System

9

Esophagus

(Sarcomas are not included.)

C15.0	Cervical esophagus	C15.4	Middle third of	C15.8	Overlapping lesion of
C15.1	Thoracic esophagus		esophagus		esophagus
C15.2	Abdominal esophagus	C15.5	Lower third of	C15.9	Esophagus, NOS
C15.3	Upper third of		esophagus		
	esophagus				

SUMMARY OF CHANGES

• The definitions of TNM and the Stage Grouping for this chapter have not changed from the Fifth Edition.

INTRODUCTION

Occurring more often in males, cancer of the esophagus accounts for 5.5% of all malignant tumors of the gastrointestinal tract and for less than 1% of all cancers in the United States. However, during the past 20 years, there has been a dramatic shift in the epidemiology of esophageal cancer in North America and most Western countries, characterized by a very rapid rise in the incidence of this disease and a marked shift from squamous cell carcinomas occurring predominantly in the middle third and distal esophagus and the esophagogastric (EG) junction. Predisposing factors for squamous cell carcinomas include a high alcohol intake and heavy use of tobacco or nutritional deficiencies of vitamins and minerals. In contrast, EG junction adenocarcinomas arise most frequently in Barrett's epithelium. The underlying causes for this marked epidemiologic change remain undefined.

Esophageal cancers, regardless of histologic type, may extend over wide areas of the mucosal surface. Squamous cell carcinomas often arise as multifocal tumors, presumably as a result of field carcinogenesis. Adenocarcinomas may have varying lengths of mucosal and submucosal disease, particularly in patients with long segments of Barrett's mucosa. However, only the depth of penetration into the esophageal wall and nodal status are considered in staging.

Many patients are asymptomatic during the early stages of disease. Early symptoms include those related to gastroesophageal reflux and associated Barrett's esophagus or odynophagia caused by esophageal ulceration. Unfortunately, the most common clinical symptom for all lesions is dysphagia, which occurs with large tumors that obstruct the lumen and deeply invade the esophageal wall. Therefore, most patients already have locally advanced or metastatic disease at diagnosis.

ANATOMY

Primary Site. Beginning at the hypopharynx, the esophagus lies posterior to the trachea and the heart, passing through the posterior mediastinum and entering the stomach through an opening in the diaphragm called the hiatus. Figure 9.1 illustrates the anatomical subsites of the esophagus, including the average measurement of each region from the incisors (front teeth).

Histologically, the esophagus has four layers: mucosa, submucosal, muscle coat or muscularis propria, and adventitia. There is no serosa.

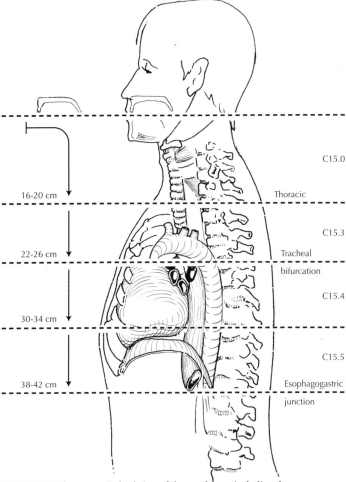

FIGURE 9.1. The anatomical subsites of the esophagus, including the average measurement of each region from the incisors. The exact measurement is body size/height dependent.

For classification, staging, and reporting of cancer, the esophagus is divided into four regions. Because the behavior of esophageal cancer and its treatment vary with the anatomic divisions, these regions should be recorded and reported separately. The location of esophageal cancer at the time of endoscopy is often measured from the incisors (front teeth).

Cervical Esophagus. The cervical esophagus begins at the level of the lower border of the cricoid cartilage and ends at the thoracic inlet (the suprasternal notch), approximately 18 cm from the upper incisor teeth.

Intrathoracic and Abdominal Esophagus. This region is divided into two portions: The *upper thoracic portion* extends from the thoracic inlet to the level of the tracheal bifurcation, approximately 24 cm from the upper incisor teeth. The *midthoracic portion* of the esophagus lies between the tracheal bifurcation and the distal esophagus just above the esophagogastric junction. The lower level of this portion is approximately 32 cm from the upper incisor teeth.

Lower Thoracic and Abdominal Portion. Approximately 3 cm in length, the lower esophagus also includes the intraabdominal portion of the esophagus and the EG junction, which is located approximately 40 cm from the upper incisor teeth. Most adenocarcinomas arise from the EG junction and involve both the distal esophagus and the proximal stomach. Controversy exists over how to distinguish proximal gastric cancers involving the EG junction from distal esophageal and EG junction adenocarcinomas extending inferiorly to involve the gastric cardia. In the absence of underlying Barrett's mucosa, making this distinction can be difficult. Siewert has proposed classifying EG junction cancers into types I, II, and III, depending on the relative extent of involvement of either the esophagus or the stomach. Further validation of this classification is needed to determine whether it is reliable for staging or for prognosis. In clinical practice, tumors arising within the EG junction and gastric cardia that have minimal (2 cm or less) involvement of the esophagus are considered primary gastric cancers.

Regional Lymph Nodes. Figure 9.2 illustrates the regional lymph nodes of the esophagus. Specific regional lymph nodes are listed as follows:

9

> Cervical esophagus
>> Scalene
>> Internal jugular
>> Upper and lower cervical
>> Periesophageal
>> Supraclavicular
>
> Intrathoracic esophagus—upper, middle, and lower
>> Upper periesophageal (above the azygous vein)
>> Subcarinal
>> Lower periesophageal (below the azygous vein)

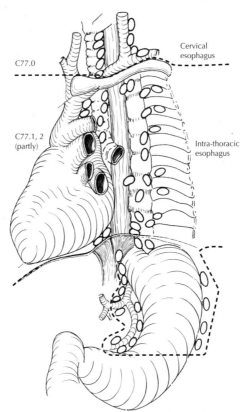

Cervical
esophagus

C77.0

C77.1, 2
(partly)

Intra-thoracic
esophagus

FIGURE 9.2. For intrathoracic tumors involvement of more distant lymph nodes (such as cervical or celiac axis nodes) is currently considered distant metastasis (M1a).

Gastroesophageal junction
    Lower esophageal (below the azygous vein)
    Diaphragmatic
    Pericardial
    Left gastric
    Celiac

Involvement of more distant lymph nodes (such as cervical or celiac axis nodes for intrathoracic tumors) is currently considered distant metastasis (M1a). However, recent analyses suggest that extensive nodal disease is associated with a better overall survival than visceral metastases and with an approximately 10% chance of cure at 5 years after surgical resection. On this basis, it has been suggested that the involvement of distant lymph nodes be classified as

N2 disease rather than M1a, but such a change in classification requires further study.

The nomenclature used to indicate the location of involved lymph nodes has most frequently been that shown above, which provides a general anatomical description. More recently, a lymph node map that extends the nomenclature and numbering system used for the staging of non–small cell lung cancer has been developed and used in clinical trials. This map, which is shown in Figure 9.1, makes possible the more precise identification of involved lymph nodes.

Metastatic Sites. The liver, lungs, and pleura are the most common sites of distant metastases. Occasionally, the tumor may extend directly into mediastinal structures before distant metastasis is evident. This occurs most frequently with tumors of the intrathoracic esophagus, which may extend directly into the aorta, trachea, and pericardium.

DEFINITIONS

Primary Tumor (T)

TX	Primary tumor cannot be assessed
T0	No evidence of primary tumor
Tis	Carcinoma *in situ*
T1	Tumor invades lamina propria or submucosal (Figure 9.3)
T2	Tumor invades muscularis propria (Figure 9.3)
T3	Tumor invades adventitia (Figure 9.4)
T4	Tumor invades adjacent structures (Figure 9.5)

Regional Lymph Nodes (N)

NX	Regional lymph nodes cannot be assessed
N0	No regional lymph node metastasis
N1	Regional lymph node metastasis (Figures 9.6, 9.7, 9.8, 9.9)

Distant Metastasis (M)

MX	Distant metastasis cannot be assessed
M0	No distant metastasis
M1	Distant metastasis (Figure 9.6)

Tumors of the lower thoracic esophagus:

M1a	Metastasis in celiac lymph nodes (Figure 9.7)
M1b	Other distant metastasis (Figure 9.7)

Tumors of the midthoracic esophagus:

M1a	Not applicable
M1b	Nonregional lymph nodes and/or other distant metastasis (Figure 9.8)

Tumors of the upper thoracic esophagus:

M1a	Metastasis in cervical nodes (Figure 9.9)
M1b	Other distant metastasis (Figure 9.9)

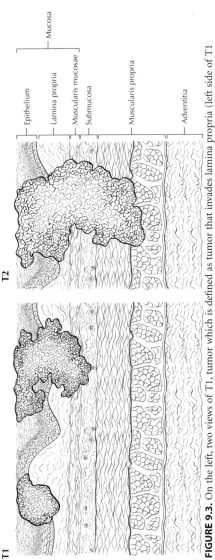

FIGURE 9.3. On the left, two views of T1, tumor which is defined as tumor that invades lamina propria (left side of T1 illustration) or submucosa (right side of T1 illustration). T2 tumor invades muscularis propria as illustrated on the right.

T3

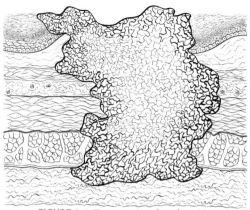

FIGURE 9.4. T3 tumor invades adventitia.

T4

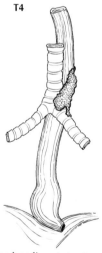

Figure 9.5. T4 tumor that invades adjacent structures (tracheobronchial involvement is shown).

9

Carcinoma of Cervical Esophagus

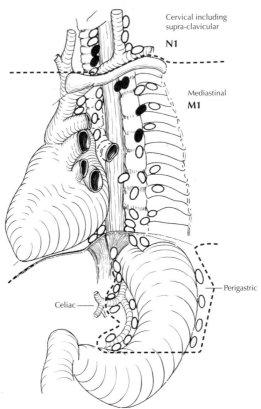

Figure 9.6. For carcinomas of the cervical esophagus, lymph node involvement outside the cervical and supraclavicular region, as illustrated here in the mediastinal region, is defined as M1 disease.

Carcinoma of Lower Thoracic Esophagus

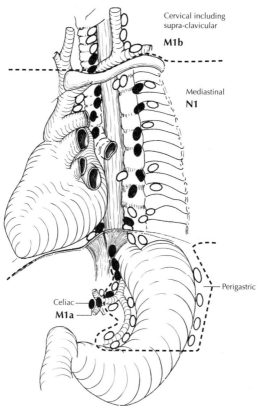

Figure 9.7. Lymph node involvement outside the regional lymph nodes of the lower thoracic esophagus, as illustrated here, is defined as M1a for metastasis in celiac lymph nodes and M1b for other distant metastasis.

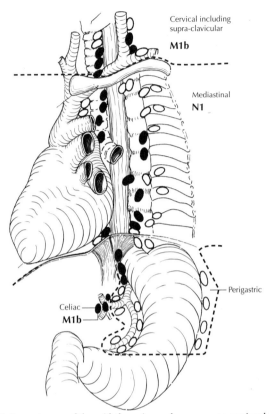

Figure 9.8. In carcinoma of the mid-thoracic esophagus, any nonregional lymph node involvement and/or other distant metastasis is defined as M1b disease.

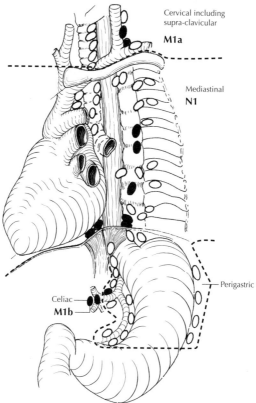

Figure 9.9. Lymph node involvement outside the regional lymph nodes of the upper thoracic esophagus, as illustrated here, is defined as M1a for metastasis in cervical lymph nodes and M1b for other distant metastasis.

STAGE GROUPING

0	Tis	N0	M0
I	T1	N0	M0
IIA	T2	N0	M0
	T3	N0	M0
IIB	T1	N1	M0
	T2	N1	M0
III	T3	N1	M0
	T4	Any N	M0
IV	Any T	Any N	M1
IVA	Any T	Any N	M1a
IVB	Any T	Any N	M1b

Stomach

(Lymphomas, sarcomas, and carcinoid tumors are not included.)

C16.0	Cardia, NOS	C16.5	Lesser curvature of the stomach, NOS	C16.8	Overlapping lesion of stomach
C16.1	Fundus of stomach				
C16.2	Body of stomach	C16.8	Greater curvature of stomach, NOS	C16.9	Stomach, NOS
C16.3	Gastric antrum				
C16.4	Pylorus				

SUMMARY OF CHANGES

- T2 lesions have been divided into T2a and T2b.
- T2a is defined as a tumor that invades the muscularis propria.
- T2b is defined as a tumor that invades into subserosa.

INTRODUCTION

Gastric adenocarcinoma has declined significantly in the United States over the past 70 years, but even so, during the early twenty-first century, an estimated 22,000 patients develop the disease each year. Of these patients, 13,000 die, mainly because of nodal and metastatic disease present at the time of initial diagnosis. When worldwide figures are analyzed, the United States ranks forty-fourth in both male and female death rates from gastric adenocarcinoma. The highest rates of this disease continue to be in areas of Asia and Russia. Trends in survival rates from the 1970s to the 1990s have unfortunately shown very little improvement. During the 1990s, 20% of gastric carcinoma cases were diagnosed while localized to the gastric wall, whereas 30% had evidence of regional nodal disease. Disease resulting from metastasis to other solid organs within the abdomen, as well as to extra-abdominal sites, represents 35% of all cases. Although overall 5-year survival is approximately 15–20%, the 5-year survival is approximately 55% when disease is localized to the stomach. The involvement of regional nodes reduces the 5-year survival to approximately 20%.

A notable shift in the site of gastric cancer reflects a proportionate increase in disease of the proximal stomach over the past several decades. Previously, there was a predominance of distal gastric cancers presenting as mass lesions or ulceration. Although other malignancies occur in the stomach, approximately 90% of all gastric neoplasms are adenocarcinomas. Tumors of the gastroe-sophageal (GE) junction may be difficult to stage as either a gastric or an esophageal primary, especially in view of the increased incidence of adenocar-cinoma in the esophagus that presumably results from acid reflux disease. By convention, if more than 50% of the cancer involves the esophagus, the cancer is classified as esophageal. Similarly, if more than 50% of the tumor is below the GE junction, it is classified as gastric in origin. If the tumor is located equally above and below the GE junction, the histology determines the origin of the primary—squamous cell, small cell, and undifferentiated carcinomas are classified as esophageal, and adenocarcinoma and signet ring cell carcinoma are classified as gastric. When Barrett's esophagus (internal metaplasia) is present, adenocarcinoma in both the gastric cardia and lower esophagus is most likely to be esophageal in origin.

ANATOMY

Primary Site. The anatomic subsites of the stomach are illustrated in Figure 10.1. The stomach is the first division of the abdominal portion of the alimentary tract, beginning at the gastroesophageal junction and extending to the pylorus. The proximal stomach is located immediately below the diaphragm and is termed the cardia. The remaining portions are the fundus (body) of the stomach and the distal portion of the stomach known as the antrum. The pylorus is a muscular ring that controls the flow of food content from the stomach into the first portion of the duodenum. The medial and lateral curvatures of the stomach are known as the lesser and greater curvatures, respectively. Histologically, the wall of the stomach has five layers: mucosal, submucosal, muscular, subserosal, and serosal.

Staging of primary gastric adenocarcinoma is dependent on the depth of penetration of the primary tumor. The T2 designation has been subdivided into T2a (invasion of the muscularis propria) and T2b (invasion of the subserosa) in order to discriminate between these intramural locations, even though there is no change in the designation in the stage grouping that involves T2a or T2b lesions.

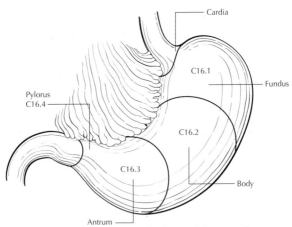

FIGURE 10.1. Anatomical subsites of the stomach.

Regional Lymph Nodes of the Stomach.

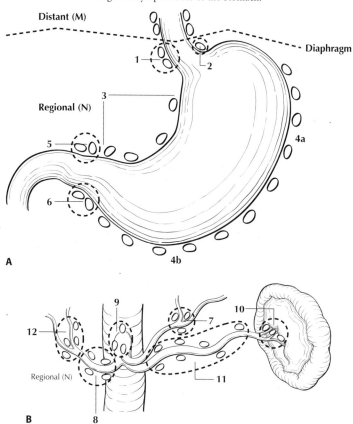

FIGURE 10.2. A. 1, 3, 5: perigastric nodes of the lesser curvature. 2, 4a, 4b, 6: perigastric nodes along the greater curvature. Involvement of nodes above the diaphragm is defined as distant metastasis. **B.** Regional lymph nodes of the stomach. 7: left gastric nodes; 8: nodes along the common hepatic artery; 9: nodes along the celiac artery; 10 and 11: nodes along the splenic artery; 12: hepatoduodenal nodes.

Regional Lymph Nodes. The regional lymph nodes of the stomach are illustrated in Figures 10.2A, B. Several groups of regional lymph nodes drain the wall of the stomach. These perigastric nodes are found along the lesser and greater curvatures. Other major nodal groups follow the main arterial and venous vessels from the aorta and portal circulation. Adequate nodal dissection of these regional nodal areas is important to ensure appropriate designation of the pN determination. Although it is suggested that at least 15 regional nodes be assessed pathologically, a pN0 determination may be assigned on the basis of the actual number of nodes evaluated microscopically.

10

Involvement of other intra-abdominal lymph nodes, such as the hepato-duodenal, retropancreatic, mesenteric, and para-aortic, is classified as distant metastasis. The specific nodal areas are as follows:

Greater Curvature of the Stomach:

Greater curvature, greater omental, gastroduodenal, gastroepiploic, pyloric, and pancreaticoduodenal

Pancreatic and Splenic Area:

Pancreaticolienal, peripancreatic, splenic

Lesser Curvature of the Stomach:

Lesser curvature, lesser omental, left gastric, cardioesophageal, common hepatic, celiac, and hepatoduodenal

Distant Nodal Groups:

Retropancreatic, para-aortic, portal, retroperitoneal, mesenteric

Metastatic Sites. The most common metastatic distribution is to the liver, peritoneal surfaces, and nonregional or distant lymph nodes. Central nervous system and pulmonary metastases occur but are less frequent. With large, bulky lesions, direct extension may occur to the liver, transverse colon, pancreas, or undersurface of the diaphragm.

DEFINITIONS

Primary Tumor (T)
TX Primary tumor cannot be assessed
T0 No evidence of primary tumor
Tis Carcinoma *in situ*: intraepithelial tumor without invasion of the lamina propria
T1 Tumor invades lamina propria or submucosa (Figure 10.3)
T2 Tumor invades muscularis propria or subserosa (Figures 10.4A, B)
T2a Tumor invades muscularis propria (Figure 10.3)
T2b Tumor invades subserosa (Figure 10.3)
T3 Tumor penetrates serosa (visceral peritoneum) without invasion of adjacent structures (Figures 10.5A, B, 10.6)
T4 Tumor invades adjacent structures (Figure 10.6)

Regional Lymph Nodes (N)
NX Regional lymph node(s) cannot be assessed
N0 No regional lymph node metastasis
N1 Metastasis in 1 to 6 regional lymph nodes (Figure 10.7)
N2 Metastasis in 7 to 15 regional lymph nodes (Figure 10.8)
N3 Metastasis in more than 15 regional lymph nodes (Figure 10.9)

Distant Metastasis (M)
MX Distant metastasis cannot be assessed
M0 No distant metastasis
M1 Distant metastasis (Figure 10.10)

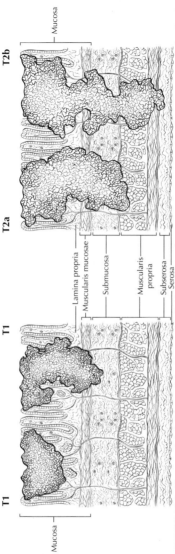

FIGURE 10.3. Illustrated definitions of T1, T2a, and T2b. Two views of T1 tumor: tumor invading lamina propria (left side of T1 illustration) and submucosa (right side of T1 illustration). T2a tumor invades muscularis propria whereas T2b tumor invades subserosa.

10

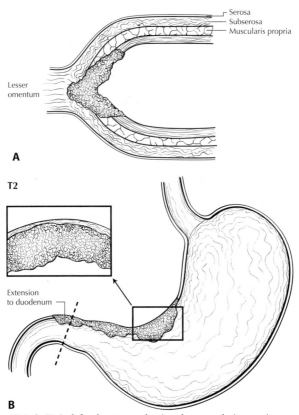

Figure 10.4. A. T2 is defined as tumor that invades muscularis propria or subserosa. **B.** T2 is defined as tumor that invades muscularis propria or subserosa. Distal extension to duodenum does not affect T category.

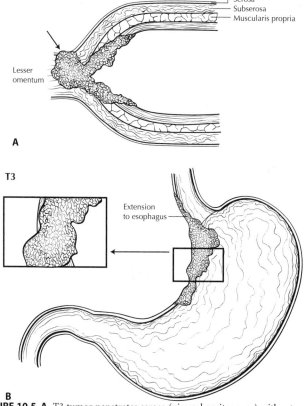

T3

Serosa
Subserosa
Muscularis propria

Lesser
omentum

A

T3

Extension
to esophagus

B

FIGURE 10.5. A. T3 tumor penetrates serosa (visceral peritoneum) without invasion of adjacent structures. **B.** T3 tumor penetrates serosa (visceral peritoneum) without invasion of adjacent structures. Proximal extension to esophagus does not affect T category.

10

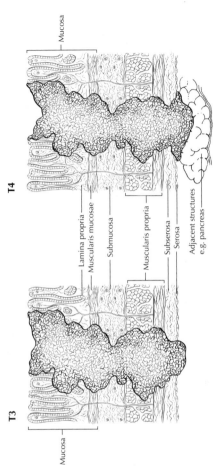

Figure 10.6. T3 tumor penetrates serosa (visceral peritoneum) without invasion of adjacent structures whereas T4 tumor radially invades adjacent structures, here the pancreas.

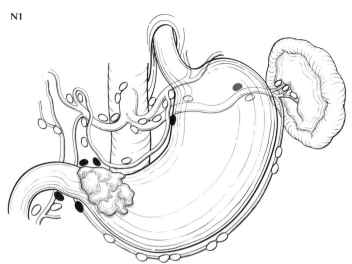

FIGURE 10.7. N1 is defined as metastasis in 1 to 6 regional lymph nodes.

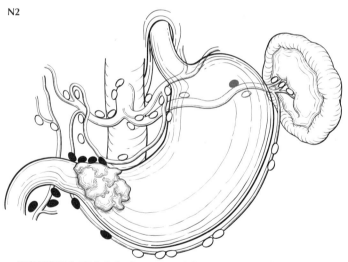

FIGURE 10.8. N2 is defined as metastasis in 7 to 15 regional lymph nodes.

10

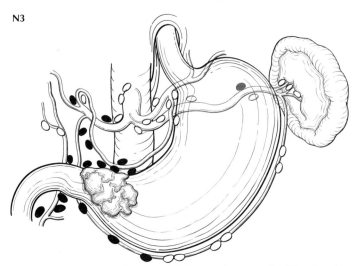

FIGURE 10.9. N3 is defined as metastasis in more than 15 regional lymph nodes.

M1

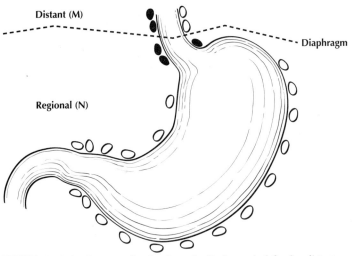

FIGURE 10.10. Involvement of nodes above the diaphragm is defined as distant metastasis or M1.

STAGE GROUPING

0	Tis	N0	M0
IA	T1	N0	M0
IB	T1	N1	M0
	T2a/b	N0	M0
II	T1	N2	M0
	T2a/b	N1	M0
	T3	N0	M0
IIIA	T2a/b	N2	M0
	T3	N1	M0
	T4	N0	M0
IIIB	T3	N2	M0
IV	T4	N1–3	M0
	T1–3	N3	M0
	Any T	Any N	M1

10

Small Intestine

(Lymphomas, carcinoid tumors, and visceral sarcomas are not included.)

C17.0	Duodenum	C17.8	Overlapping lesion of	C17.9	Small intestine,
C17.1	Jejunum		small intestine		NOS
C17.2	Ileum				

SUMMARY OF CHANGES

• The definitions of TNM and the Stage Grouping for this chapter have not changed from the Fifth Edition.

INTRODUCTION

Although the small intestine accounts for one of the largest surface areas in the human body, less than 2% of all malignant tumors of the gastrointestinal tract actually occur in the small bowel. Most cancers occur in the first or second portion of the duodenum and are adenocarcinomas. A variety of other tumor types occur in the small intestine, but approximately 50% of the primary malignant tumors are adenocarcinomas. An increased incidence of second malignancies has been noted in patients with primary small bowel adenocarcinoma. At the beginning of the twenty-first century, approximately 5,000 new cases of cancer involving the small intestine are seen annually in the United States. The 1,200 deaths predicted to occur from small intestinal cancer are divided equally between men and women. The patterns of local, regional, and metastatic spread for adenocarcinomas of the small intestine are comparable to those of similar histologic malignancies in other areas of the gastrointestinal tract. The classification and stage groupings described in this chapter are used for both clinical and pathologic staging of carcinomas of the small bowel and do not apply to other types of malignant small bowel tumors. Although small bowel carcinoid tumors are not traditionally staged using the TNM system, reports from the United States and throughout the world attempt to stage these neuroendocrine tumors using the TNM system.

ANATOMY

Primary Site. This classification applies to carcinomas arising in the duodenum, jejunum, and ileum. These anatomical sites are illustrated in Figure 11.1. It does not apply to carcinomas arising in the ileocecal valve or to carcinomas that may arise in Meckel's diverticulum. Carcinomas arising in the ampulla of Vater are staged according to the system described in Chapter 17.

Duodenum. About 25 cm in length, the duodenum extends from the pyloric sphincter of the stomach to the jejunum. It is usually divided anatomically into four parts, with the common bile duct and pancreatic duct opening into the second part at the ampulla of Vater.

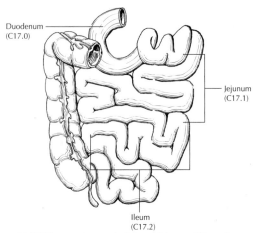

FIGURE 11.1. Anatomical sites of the small intestine.

Jejunum and Ileum. The jejunum (8 feet in length) and ileum (12 feet in length) extend from the junction with the duodenum proximally to the ileocecal valve distally. The division point between the jejunum and the ileum is arbitrary. As a general rule, the jejunum includes the proximal 40% and the ileum includes the distal 60% of the small intestine, exclusive of the duodenum.

General. The jejunal and ileal portions of the small intestine are supported by the mesentery, which is a fold of the peritoneum containing the blood supply and the regional lymph nodes. The shortest segment, the duodenum, has no real mesentery and is covered by peritoneum only over its anterior surface. The wall of all parts of the small intestine has five layers: mucosal, submucosal, muscular, subserosal, and serosal. A very thin layer of smooth muscle cells, the muscularis mucosae, separates the mucosa from the submucosal. The small intestine is entirely ensheathed by peritoneum, except for a narrow strip of bowel that is attached to the mesentery and that part of the duodenum that is located retroperitoneally.

Regional Lymph Nodes. For pN, histologic examination of a regional lymphadenectomy specimen will ordinarily include a representative number of lymph nodes distributed along the mesenteric vessels extending to the base of the mesentery.

Duodenum:
Duodenal
Hepatic
Pancreaticoduodenal
Infrapyloric
Gastroduodenal
Pyloric
Superior mesenteric

Pericholedochal
Regional lymph nodes, NOS

Ileum and Jejunum:
Posterior cecal (terminal ileum only)
Ileocolic (terminal ileum only)
Superior mesenteric
Mesenteric, NOS
Regional lymph nodes, NOS

Metastatic Sites. Cancers of the small intestine can metastasize to most organs, especially the liver, or to the peritoneal surfaces. Involvement of regional lymph nodes and invasion of adjacent structures are most common. Involvement of the celiac nodes is considered M1 disease for carcinomas of the duodenum, jejunum, and ileum. The presence of distant metastases and the presence of residual disease (R) have the most influence on survival.

DEFINITIONS

Primary Tumor (T)

TX	Primary tumor cannot be assessed
T0	No evidence of primary tumor
Tis	Carcinoma *in situ*
T1	Tumor invades lamina propria or submucosal (Figure 11.2)
T2	Tumor invades muscularis propria (Figure 11.3)
T3	Tumor invades through the muscularis propria into the subserosa (Figure 11.4, top) or into the nonperitonealized perimuscular tissue (mesentery or retroperitoneum) with extension 2 cm or less[1] (Figures 11.5, top)
T4	Tumor perforates the visceral peritoneum (Figure 11.4, bottom) or directly invades other organs or structures (includes mesentery, or retroperitoneum more than 2 cm [Figure 11.5, bottom], other loops of small intestine [Figure 11.6], and abdominal wall by way of serosa; for duodenum only, invasion of pancreas [Figure 11.7])

T1

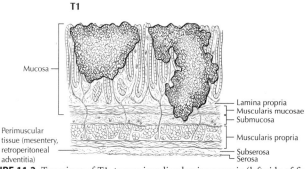

FIGURE 11.2. Two views of T1: tumor invading lamina propria (left side of figure) or submucosa (right side of figure).

11

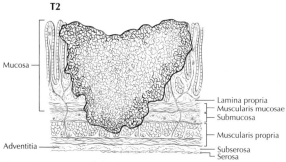

FIGURE 11.3. T2 is defined as tumor invading muscularis propria.

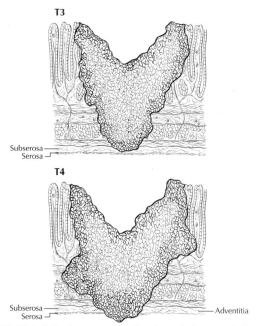

FIGURE 11.4. T3 is defined as tumor invading through the muscularis propria into the subserosa whereas T4 is defined as tumor that perforates (penetrates) the visceral peritoneum.

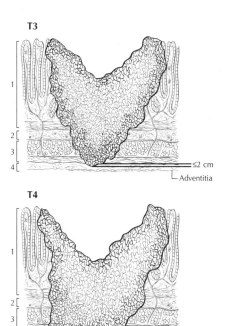

T3

T4

1 Mucosa
2 Submucosa
3 Muscularis propria
4 Perimuscular tissue (mesentery, retroperitoneal
  adventitia, or subserosa)

FIGURE 11.5. T3 is defined as tumor invading into the nonperitonealized perimuscular tissue (mesentery or retroperitoneum) with extension 2 cm or less whereas T4 directly invades other organs or structures (includes, mesentery, or retroperitoneum) more than 2 cm.

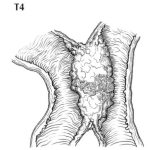

T4

FIGURE 11.6. T4 directly invades other organs or structures, including other loops of small intestine.

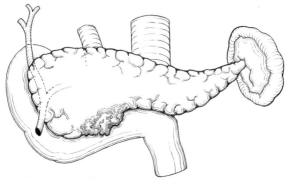

FIGURE 11.7. T4 (duodenum only) tumor invades the pancreas.

Regional Lymph Nodes (N)

NX Regional lymph nodes cannot be assessed
N0 No regional lymph node metastasis
N1 Regional lymph node metastasis

Distant Metastasis (M)

MX Distant metastasis cannot be assessed
M0 No distant metastasis
M1 Distant metastasis

STAGE GROUPING

0	Tis	N0	M0
I	T1	N0	M0
	T2	N0	M0
II	T3	N0	M0
	T4	N0	M0
III	Any T	N1	M0
IV	Any T	Any N	M1

NOTE

1. The nonperitonealized perimuscular tissue is, for jejunum and ileum, part of the mesentery and, for duodenum in areas where serosa is lacking, part of the retroperitoneum.

Colon and Rectum

(Sarcomas, lymphomas, and carcinoid tumors of the large intestine or appendix are not included.)

C18.0	Cecum	C18.5	Splenic flexure of colon	C18.9	Colon, NOS
C18.1	Appendix			C19.9	Rectosigmoid
C18.2	Ascending colon	C18.6	Descending colon		junction
C18.3	Hepatic flexure of colon	C18.7	Sigmoid colon	C20.9	Rectum, NOS
C18.4	Transverse colon	C18.8	Overlapping lesion of colon		

SUMMARY OF CHANGES

- A revised description of the anatomy of the colon and rectum better delineates the data concerning the boundaries between colon, rectum, and anal canal. Adenocarcinomas of the vermiform appendix are classified according to the TNM staging system but should be recorded separately, whereas cancers that occur in the anal canal are staged according to the classification used for the anus.

- Smooth extramural nodules of any size in the pericolic or perirectal fat are considered lymph node metastases and will be counted in the N staging. In contrast, irregularly contoured nodules in the peritumoral fat are considered vascular invasion and will be coded as transmural extension in the T category and further denoted as either a V1 (microscopic vascular invasion) if only microscopically visible or a V2 (macroscopic vascular invasion) if grossly visible.

- Stage Group II is subdivided into IIA and IIB on the basis of whether the primary tumor is T3 or T4 respectively.

- Stage Group III is subdivided into IIIA (T1-2N1M0), IIIB (T3-4N1M0), or IIIC (any TN2M0).

INTRODUCTION

The TNM classification for carcinomas of the colon and rectum provides more detail than other staging systems. Compatible with the Dukes' system, the TNM adds greater precision in the identification of prognostic subgroups. TNM staging is based on the depth of tumor invasion into the wall of the intestine (T), extension to adjacent structures (T), the number of regional lymph nodes involved (N), and the presence or absence of distant metastasis (M). The TNM classification applies to both clinical and pathologic staging. However, most cancers of the colon or rectum are staged after pathologic examination of the surgical resection specimen. This staging system applies to all carcinomas arising in the colon or rectum. Adenocarcinomas of the vermiform appendix may be classified according to the TNM staging system but should be recorded separately. Since stage-specific outcomes may differ from colorectal carcinomas. Cancers that occur in the anal canal are staged according to the classification used for the anus (see Chapter 13).

12

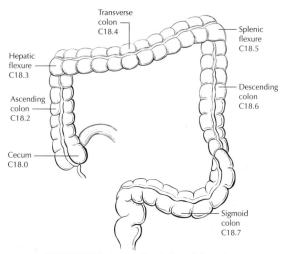

FIGURE 12.1. Anatomic subsites of the colon.

ANATOMY

The anatomical subsites of the colon and rectum are illustrated in Figures 12.1 and 12.2, respectively. The divisions of the colon and rectum are as follows:

Cecum
Ascending colon
Hepatic flexure
Transverse colon
Splenic flexure
Descending colon
Sigmoid colon

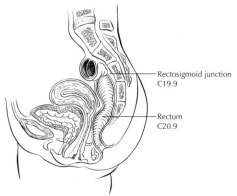

FIGURE 12.2. Anatomic subsites of the rectum.

American Joint Committee on Cancer • 2006

Rectosigmoid colon
Rectum

Primary Site. The large intestine (colorectum) extends from the terminal ileum to the anal canal. Excluding the rectum and vermiform appendix, the colon is divided into four parts: the right or ascending colon, the middle or transverse colon, the left or descending colon, and the sigmoid colon. The sigmoid is continuous with the rectum, which terminates at the anal canal.

The cecum is a large, blind pouch that arises from the proximal segment of the right colon. It measures 6 cm by 9 cm and is covered with peritoneum. The ascending colon measures 15–20 cm in length. The posterior surface of the ascending (and descending) colon lacks peritoneum and thus is in direct contact with the retroperitoneum. In contrast, the anterior and lateral surfaces of the ascending (and descending) colon have serosa and are intraperitoneal. The hepatic flexure connects the ascending colon with the transverse colon, passing just inferior to the liver and anterior to the duodenum.

The transverse colon is entirely intraperitoneal, supported on a long mesentery that is attached to the pancreas. Anteriorly, its serosa is continuous with the gastrocolic ligament. The splenic flexure connects the transverse colon to the descending colon, passing inferior to the spleen and anterior to the tail of the pancreas. As noted above, the posterior aspect of the descending colon lacks serosa and is in direct contact with the retroperitoneum, whereas the lateral and anterior surfaces have serosa and are intraperitoneal. The descending colon measures 10–15 cm in length. The colon becomes completely intraperitoneal once again at the sigmoid colon, where the mesentery develops at the medial border of the left posterior major psoas muscle and extends to the rectum. The transition from sigmoid colon to rectum is marked by the fusion of the tenia of the sigmoid colon to form the circumferential longitudinal muscle of the rectum. This occurs roughly 12–15 cm from the dentate line.

Approximately 12 cm in length, the rectum extends proximally from the fusion of the tenia to the puborectalis ring distally. The rectum is covered by peritoneum in front and on both sides in its upper third and only on the anterior wall in its middle third. The peritoneum is reflected laterally from the rectum to form the perirectal fossa and, anteriorly, the uterine or rectovesical fold. There is no peritoneal covering in the lower third, which is often known as the rectal ampulla. The anal canal, which measures 3–5 cm in length, extends from the puborectalis sling to the anal verge.

Regional Lymph Nodes. Regional nodes are located (1) along the course of the major vessels supplying the colon and rectum, (2) along the vascular arcades of the marginal artery, and (3) adjacent to the colon—that is, located along the mesocolic border of the colon. Specifically, the regional lymph nodes are the pericoloic and perirectal nodes and those found along the ileocolic, right colic, middle colic, left colic, inferior mesenteric artery, superior rectal (hemorrhoidal), and internal iliac arteries (Figure 12.3).

For pN, the number of lymph nodes sampled should be recorded. The number of nodes examined from an operative specimen has been reported to be associated with improved survival, possibly because of increased accuracy in

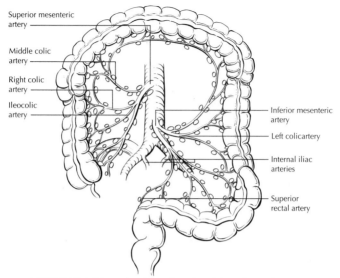

FIGURE 12.3. The regional lymph nodes of the colon and rectum.

staging. It is important to obtain at least 12–14 lymph nodes in radical colon and rectum resections; however, in cases in which tumor is resected for palliation or in patients who have received preoperative radiation, only a few lymph nodes may be present. A pN0 determination may be assessed when these nodes are histologically negative, even though fewer than the recommended number of nodes have been analyzed.

The regional lymph nodes for each segment of the large bowel are designated as follows:

Segment	*Regional Lymph Nodes*
Cecum	Pericolic, anterior cecal, posterior cecal, ileocolic, right colic
Ascending colon	Pericolic, ileocolic, right colic, middle colic
Hepatic flexure	Pericolic, middle colic, right colic
Transverse colon	Pericolic, middle colic
Splenic flexure	Pericolic, middle colic, left colic, inferior mesenteric
Descending colon	Pericolic, left colic, inferior mesenteric, sigmoid
Sigmoid colon	Pericolic, inferior mesenteric, superior rectal (hemorrhoidal), sigmoidal, sigmoid mesenteric
Rectosigmoid	Pericolic, perirectal, left colic, sigmoid mesenteric, sigmoidal, inferior mesenteric, superior rectal (hemorrhoidal), middle rectal (hemorrhoidal)
Rectum	Perirectal, sigmoid mesenteric, inferior mesenteric, lateral sacral presacral, internal iliac, sacral promontory (Gerota's), superior rectal (hemorrhoidal), middle rectal (hemorrhoidal), inferior rectal (hemorrhoidal)

T1

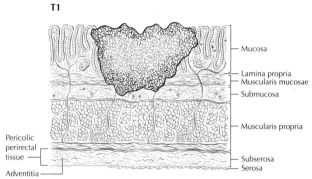

FIGURE 12.4. T1 tumor invades submucosal.

Metastatic Sites. Although carcinomas of the colon and rectum can metastasize to almost any organ, the liver and lungs are the most common sites. Seeding of other segments of the colon, small intestine, or peritoneum can also occur.

DEFINITIONS

Primary Tumor (T)

TX   Primary tumor cannot be assessed
T0   No evidence of primary tumor
Tis   Carcinoma *in situ*: intraepithelial or invasion of lamina propria[1]
T1   Tumor invades submucosa (Figure 12.4)
T2   Tumor invades muscularis propria (Figure 12.5)
T3   Tumor invades through the muscularis propria into the subserosa, or into nonperitonealized pericolic or perirectal tissues (Figure 12.6)
T4   Tumor directly invades other organs or structures (Figures 12.7A–C), and/or perforates visceral peritoneum[2,3] (Figures 12.7C, D)

T2

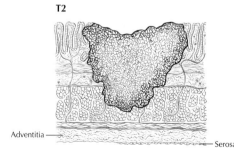

FIGURE 12.5. T2 tumor invades muscularis propria.

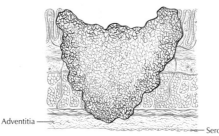

FIGURE 12.6. T3 tumor invades through the muscularis propria into the subserosa or into nonperitonealized pericolic, or perirectal tissues (adventitia).

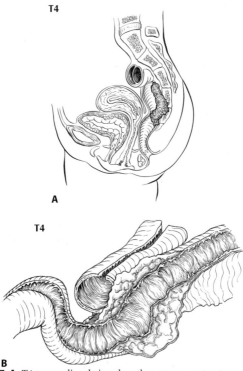

FIGURE 12.7. A. T4 tumor directly invades other organs or structures (such as the coccyx shown here), and/or perforates visceral peritoneum. **B.** T4 tumor directly invades other organs or structures, and/or perforates visceral peritoneum, as illustrated here with radial extension into an adjacent loop of small bowel.

T4

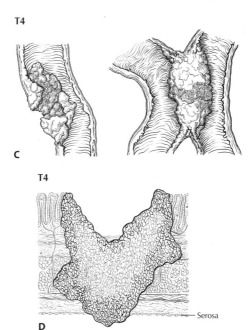

Serosa

D

FIGURE 12.7. C. T4 tumor directly invades other organs or structures (such as adjacent bowel, shown right), and/or perforates visceral peritoneum (shown left with gross bowel perforation through the tumor). **D.** T4 tumor directly invades other organs or structures, and/or perforates (penetrates) visceral peritoneum, as illustrated here.

Regional Lymph Nodes (N)

NX   Regional lymph nodes cannot be assessed[4]

N0   No regional lymph node metastasis

N1   Metastasis in 1 to 3 regional lymph nodes (Figure 12.8)

N2   Metastasis in 4 or more regional lymph nodes (Figures 12.9A–C)

Distant Metastasis (M)

MX   Distant metastasis cannot be assessed

M0   No distant metastasis

M1   Distant metastasis (Figure 12.10)

Residual Tumor (R)

R0   Complete resection, margins histologically negative, no residual tumor left after resection

R1   Incomplete resection, margins histologically involved, microscopic tumor remains after resection of gross disease.

R2   Incomplete resection, margins involved or gross disease remains after resection (Figure 12.11)

12

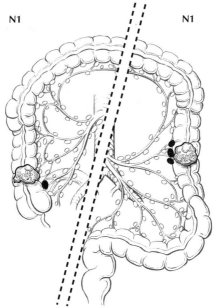

N1   N1

FIGURE 12.8. Two views of N1, which is defined as metastasis in 1 to 3 regional lymph nodes.

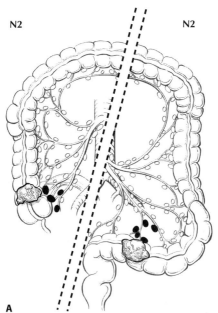

N2   N2

A

FIGURE 12.9. A. Two views of N2, which is defined as metastasis in 4 or more regional lymph nodes.

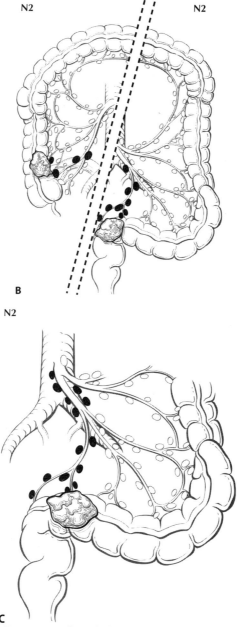

FIGURE 12.9. B. Two views of N2 which is defined as metastasis in 4 or more regional lymph nodes. **C.** N2 showing nodal masses in more than 4 regional lymph nodes.

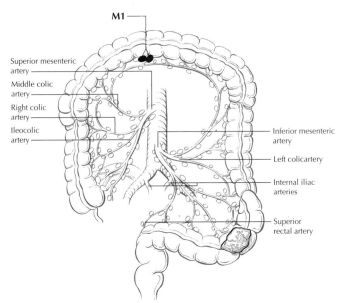

FIGURE 12.10. M1 disease is defined as distant metastasis, in this case outside the regional nodes of the primary tumor.

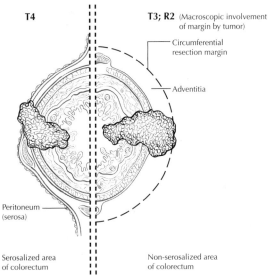

FIGURE 12.11. T4 (left side) has perforated the visceral peritoneum in a segment of the colorectum with a serosal covering. In contrast, T3; R2 (right side) shows macroscopic involvement of the circumferential resection margin of a nonperitonealized surface of the colorectum by tumor corresponds to gross disease remaining after surgical excision).

STAGE GROUPING

Stage	T	N	M	Dukes	MAC
0	Tis	N0	M0	—	—
I	T1	N0	M0	A	A
	T2	N0	M0	A	Bl
IIA	T3	N0	M0	B	B2
IIB	T4	N0	M0	B	B3
IIIA	T1–T3	N1	M0	C	Cl
IIIB	T3–T4	N1	M0	C	C2/C3
IIIC	Any T	N2	M0	C	C1/C2/C3
IV	Any T	Any N	M1	—	D

NOTES

1. Tis includes cancer cells confined within the glandular basement membrane (intraepithelial) or lamina propria (intramucosal) with no extension through the muscularis mucosae into the submucosa.
2. Direct invasion in T4 includes invasion of other segments of the colorectum by way of the serosa, for example, invasion of the sigmoid colon by a carcinoma of the cecum.
3. Tumor that is adherent to other organs or structures, macroscopically, is classified T4. However, if no tumor is present in the adhesion, microscopically, the classification should be pT3. The V and L substaging should be used to identify the presence or absence of vascular or lymphatic invasion.
4. A tumor nodule in the pericolorectal adipose tissue of a primary carcinoma without histologic evidence of residual lymph node in the nodule is classified in the pN category as a regional lymph node metastasis if the nodule has the form and smooth contour of a lymph node. If the nodule has an irregular contour, it should be classified in the T category and also coded as V1 (microscopic venous invasion) or as V2 (if it was grossly evident), because there is a strong likelihood that it represents venous invasion.

12

Anal Canal

(The classification applies to carcinomas only; melanomas, carcinoid tumors, and sarcomas are not included.)

C21.0	Anus, NOS	C21.8	Ovelapping lesion of
C21.1	Anal canal		rectum, anus, and
C21.2	Cloacogenic zone		anal canal

SUMMARY OF CHANGES

• The definitions of TNM and the Stage Groupings for this chapter have not changed from the Fifth Edition.

INTRODUCTION

The proximal region of the anus encompasses true mucosa of three different histologic types: glandular, transitional, and squamous (proximal to distal, respectively). Distally, the squamous mucosa merges with the perianal skin (true epidermis). This mucocutaneous junction historically has been called the anal verge or margin. Thus, two distinct categories of tumors arise in the anal region. Tumors that develop from mucosa (of any of the three types) are termed anal canal cancers, whereas those that arise within skin at or distal to the squamous mucocutaneous junction are termed anal margin tumors. The proximal boundary of the anal margin is indistinct on macroscopic examination and, anatomically, may vary with the patient's body habitus. A proximal boundary located 5–6 cm from the squamous mucocutaneous junction applies in the majority of adults.

Anal canal tumors are staged using the classification system described and illustrated herein. Anal margin tumors are biologically comparable to other skin tumors and therefore are classified by the schema presented in Chapter 23, Carcinoma of the Skin. However, the regional nodal drainage (relevant to the N category) of the skin of the anal margin is uniquely specific to this anatomic site, as outlined in this section.

Because the primary management of carcinomas of the anal canal has shifted from surgical resection to nonsurgical treatment, they are typically staged clinically according to the size and extent of the primary tumor. Thus, patients with cancer of the anal canal may be staged at the time of presentation by inspection, palpation and biopsy of the mass, palpation (and biopsy as needed) of regional lymph nodes, and radiologic imaging of the chest, abdomen, and pelvis.

ANATOMY

Primary Site. The anatomic subsites of the anal canal are illustrated in Figure 13.1. The anal canal begins where the rectum enters the puborectalis sling at the apex of the anal sphincter complex (palpable as the anorectal ring on digital

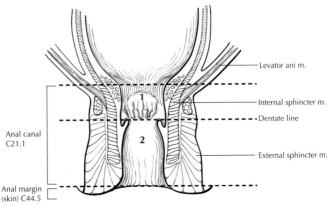

Anal canal
C21.1

Anal margin
(skin) C44.5

Levator ani m.

Internal sphincter m.

Dentate line

External sphincter m.

1. Transitional epithelium
2. Squamous epithelium devoid of hair and glands (not skin)

FIGURE 13.1. Anatomic subsites of the anal canal.

exam) and ends at the squamous mucocutaneous junction with the perianal skin. The most proximal aspect of the anal canal is lined by colorectal mucosa, and at the dentate line, a narrow zone of transitional mucosa that is similar to urothelium is variably present. The proximal zone (from the top of the puborectalis to the dentate line, including the transitional zone) measures approximately 1–2 cm. In the region of the dentate line, anal glands may be found subadjacent to the mucosa, often extending across the internal sphincter to the intersphincteric plane. A proximal boundary located distal to the dentate line and extending to the mucocutaneous junction is a nonkeratinizing squamous epithelium devoid of skin appendages (hair follicles, apocrine glands, and sweat glands).

Carcinomas that overlap the anorectal junction may be problematic. They should be staged as rectal tumors if their epicenter is located more than 2 cm proximal to the dentate line and as anal tumors if their epicenter is 2 cm or less from the dentate line. However, extension of low rectal tumors beyond the dentate line implies risk of metastatic spread to the superficial inguinal lymph nodes.

Regional Lymph Nodes. Lymphatic drainage and nodal involvement of anal cancers depend on the location of the primary tumor. Tumors above the dentate line spread primarily to the anorectal, perirectal, and paravertebral nodes, whereas tumors below the dentate line spread to the superficial inguinal nodes.

The regional lymph nodes are as follows (Figure 13.2):

Perirectal
    Anorectal
    Perirectal
    Lateral sacral
Internal iliac (hypogastric)

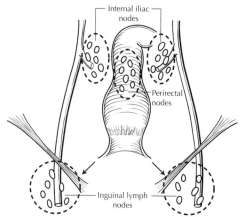

FIGURE 13.2. Regional lymph nodes of the anal canal.

Inguinal
    Superficial
    Deep femoral
All other nodal groups represent sites of distant metastasis.

Metastatic Sites. Cancers of the anus may metastasize to any organs, but the liver and lungs are the distal organs that are most frequently involved. Involvement of the abdominal cavity is not unusual.

DEFINITIONS

Primary Tumor (T)

TX   Primary tumor cannot be assessed
T0   No evidence of primary tumor
Tis   Carcinoma *in situ*
T1   Tumor 2 cm or less in greatest dimension (Figure 13.3)
T2   Tumor more than 2 cm but not more than 5 cm in greatest dimension (Figure 13.4)
T3   Tumor more than 5 cm in greatest dimension (Figure 13.5)
T4   Tumor of any size invades adjacent organ(s), e.g., vagina, urethra, bladder[1] (Figure 13.6)

Regional Lymph Nodes (N)

NX   Regional lymph nodes cannot be assessed
N0   No regional lymph node metastasis
N1   Metastasis in perirectal lymph node(s) (Figure 13.7)
N2   Metastasis in unilateral internal iliac and/or inguinal lymph node(s) (Figures 13.8A, B)
N3   Metastasis in perirectal and inguinal lymph nodes and/or bilateral internal iliac and/or inguinal lymph nodes (Figures 13.9A–C)

T1

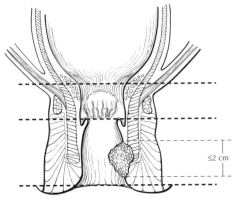

FIGURE 13.3. T1 is defined as tumor 2 cm or less in greatest dimension.

T2   **T2**

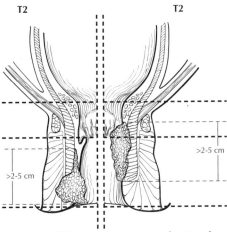

FIGURE 13.4. Two views of T2 showing tumor more than 2 cm but not more than 5 cm in greatest dimension. On the right side of the diagram, the tumor extends above the dentate line.

T3

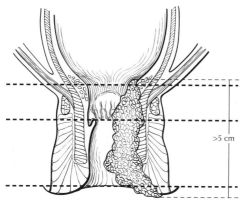

>5 cm

FIGURE 13.5. T3 is defined as tumor more than 5 cm in greatest dimension.

T4

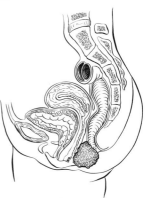

FIGURE 13.6. T4 is defined as tumor of any size invading adjacent organ(s), e.g., vagina (as illustrated), urethra, bladder.[1]

N1

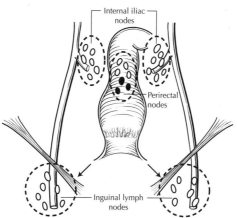

Internal iliac nodes

Perirectal nodes

Inguinal lymph nodes

FIGURE 13.7. N1 is defined as metastasis in perirectal lymph node(s).

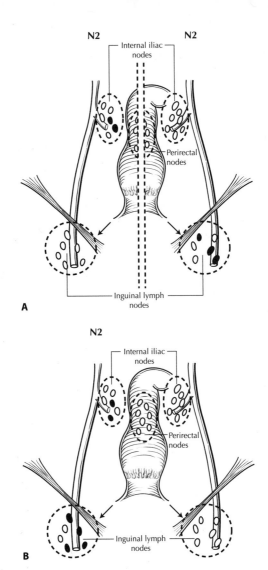

FIGURE 13.8. A. Two views of N2, which is defined as metastasis in unilateral internal iliac (left) and/or inguinal lymph node(s) (right). **B.** N2: metastases in unilateral internal iliac *and* inguinal lymph node(s).

FIGURE 13.9. A. N3 is defined as metastasis in perirectal and inguinal lymph nodes (as illustrated) and/or bilateral internal iliac and/or inguinal lymph nodes. **B.** N3: metastases in bilateral internal iliac lymph nodes. **C.** N3: metastases in bilateral internal iliac *and* inguinal lymph nodes.

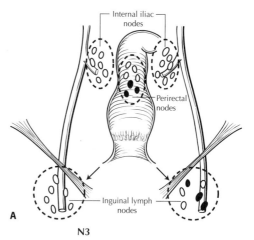

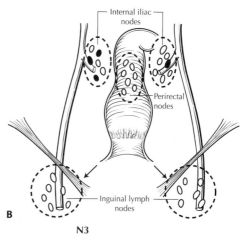

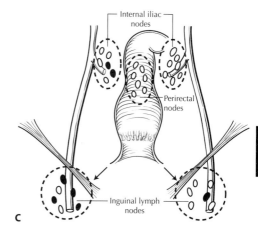

Distant Metastasis (M)

MX   Distant metastasis cannot be assessed
M0   No distant metastasis
M1   Distant metastasis

STAGE GROUPING

0	Tis	N0	M0
I	T1	N0	M0
II	T2	N0	M0
	T3	N0	M0
IIIA	T1	N1	M0
	T2	N1	M0
	T3	N1	M0
	T4	N0	M0
IIIB	T4	N1	M0
	Any T	N2	M0
	Any T	N3	M0
IV	Any T	Any N	M1

NOTE

1. Direct invasion of the rectal wall, perirectal skin, subcutaneous tissue, or the sphincter muscle(s) is not classified as T4.

Liver (Including Intrahepatic Bile Ducts)

(Sarcomas and tumors metastatic to the liver are not included.)

C22.0   Liver   C22.1   Intrahepatic bile duct

SUMMARY OF CHANGES

- The T categories in this edition have been redefined and simplified.

- All solitary tumors without vascular invasion, regardless of size, are classified as T1 because of similar prognosis.

- All solitary tumors with vascular invasion (again regardless of size) are combined with multiple tumors ≤5 cm and classified as T2 because of similar prognosis.

- Multiple tumors >5 cm and tumors with evidence of major vascular invasion are combined and classified as T3 because of similarly poor prognosis.

- Tumor(s) with direct invasion of adjacent organs other than the gallbladder or with perforation of visceral peritoneum are classified separately as T4.

- The separate subcategory for multiple bilobar tumors has been eliminated because of a lack of distinct prognostic value.

- T3 N0 tumors and tumors with lymph node involvement are combined into Stage III because of similar prognosis.

- Stage IV defines metastatic disease only. The subcategories IVA and IVB have been eliminated.

INTRODUCTION

Primary malignancies of the liver include tumors arising from the hepatocytes (hepatocellular carcinoma), intrahepatic bile ducts (intrahepatic cholangiocarcinoma and cystadenocarcinoma), and mesenchymal elements (primary sarcomas, not covered in this chapter). Hepatocellular carcinoma is the most common primary cancer of the liver and is a leading cause of death from cancer worldwide. Although it is uncommon in the United States, its incidence is rising. The majority of hepatocellular carcinomas arise in a background of chronic liver disease due to viral hepatitis (B or C) or ethanol abuse. Cirrhosis may dominate the clinical picture and determine the prognosis. Other important indicators of the outcome of hepatocellular carcinoma are resectability for cure and the extent of vascular invasion.

ANATOMY

Primary Site. The liver has a dual blood supply: the hepatic artery, which branches from the celiac artery, and the portal vein, which drains the intestine. Blood from the liver passes through the hepatic vein and enters the inferior vena cava. The liver is divided into right and left lobes by a plane (Cantlie's line) projecting between the gallbladder fossa and the vena cava and defined by the

---

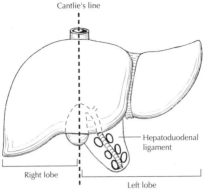

FIGURE 14.1. Division of the liver into right and left lobes by the plane of Cantlie's line.

middle hepatic vein (Figure 14.1). Couinaud refined knowledge about the functional anatomy of the liver and proposed division of the liver into four sectors (formerly called segments) and eight segments. In this nomenclature, the liver is divided by vertical and oblique planes or scissurae defined by the three main hepatic veins and a transverse plane or scissura that follows a line drawn through the right and left portal branches. Thus, the four traditional segments (right anterior, right posterior, left medial, and left lateral) are replaced by sectors (right anterior, right posterior, left anterior, and left posterior), and these sectors are divided into segments by the transverse scissura (Figure 14.2). The eight segments are numbered clockwise in a frontal plane. Recent advances in hepatic

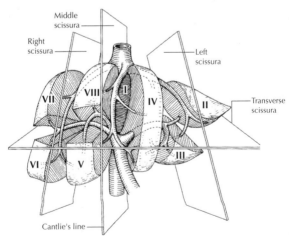

FIGURE 14.2. Anatomy of the liver.

surgery have made possible anatomic (also called typical) resections along these planes.

Histologically, the liver is divided into lobules with central veins draining each lobule. The portal spaces between the lobules contain the intrahepatic bile ducts and the blood supply, which consists of small branches of the hepatic artery and portal vein (portal triads).

Regional Lymph Nodes. The regional lymph nodes are the hilar, hepatoduodenal ligament lymph nodes, and caval lymph nodes, among which the most prominent are the hepatic artery and portal vein lymph nodes. Histologic examination of a regional lymphadenectomy specimen will ordinarily include a minimum of three lymph nodes.

Nodal involvement beyond these lymph nodes is considered distant metastasis and should be coded as M1. Involvement of the inferior phrenic lymph nodes should also be considered M1.

Metastatic Sites. The main mode of dissemination of liver carcinomas is via the portal veins (intrahepatic) and hepatic veins. Intrahepatic venous dissemination cannot be differentiated from satellitosis or multifocal tumors and is classified as multiple tumors. The most common sites of extrahepatic dissemination are the lungs and bones. Tumors may extend through the liver capsule to adjacent organs (adrenal, diaphragm, and colon) or may rupture, causing acute hemorrhage and peritoneal carcinomatosis.

DEFINITIONS

Primary Tumor (T)

TX   Primary tumor cannot be assessed
T0   No evidence of primary tumor
T1   Solitary tumor without vascular invasion (Figure 14.3)
T2   Solitary tumor with vascular invasion or multiple tumors, none more than 5 cm (Figures 14.4A, B)

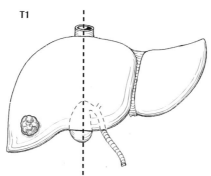

FIGURE 14.3. T1 is defined as a solid tumor without vascular invasion, regardless of size.

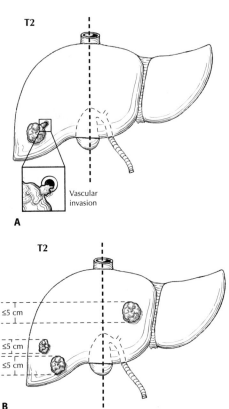

T2

Vascular invasion

A

T2

≤5 cm

≤5 cm

≤5 cm

B

FIGURE 14.4. A. All solitary tumors with vascular invasion, regardless of size, are classified T2. **B.** Multiple tumors, with none more than 5 cm, are classified T2.

T3   Multiple tumors more than 5 cm or tumor involving a major branch of the portal or hepatic vein(s) (Figures 14.5A, B)

T4   Tumor(s) with direct invasion of adjacent organs other than the gallbladder or with perforation of visceral peritoneum (Figure 14.6)

Regional Lymph Nodes (N)
NX   Regional lymph nodes cannot be assessed
N0   No regional lymph node metastasis
N1   Regional lymph node metastasis (Figure 14.7)

Distant Metastasis (M)
MX   Distant metastasis cannot be assessed
M0   No distant metastasis
M1   Distant metastasis

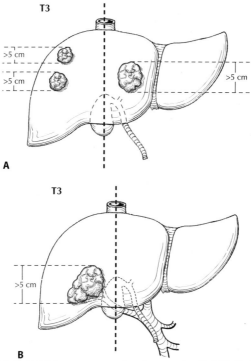

FIGURE 14.5. A. Multiple tumors more than 5 cm are classified T3. **B.** A tumor involving a major branch of the portal or hepatic vein(s) is classified T3.

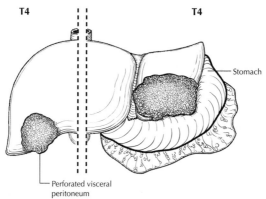

FIGURE 14.6. Two views of T4: tumor with perforation of the visceral peritoneum(left of dotted line); tumor directly invading adjacent organs other than the gallbladder (right of dotted line, tumor invades stomach).

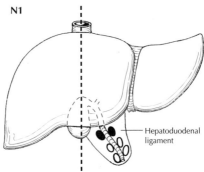

FIGURE 14.7. N1 is defined as metastasis to regional lymph nodes.

STAGE GROUPING

I	T1	N0	M0
II	T2	N0	M0
IIIA	T3	N0	M0
IIIB	T4	N0	M0
IIIC	Any T	N1	M0
IV	Any T	Any N	M1

15

Gallbladder

(Carcinoid tumors and sarcomas are not included.)

15

C23.9   Gallbladder

SUMMARY OF CHANGES

- The T and N classifications have been simplified in an effort to separate locally invasive tumors into potentially resectable (T3) and unresectable (T4).

- There is no longer a distinction between T3 and T4 based on the depth of liver invasion.

- Lymph node metastasis is now classified as Stage IIB, and Stage IIA is reserved for large, invasive tumors (resectable), without lymph node metastasis.

- Stage grouping has been changed to allow Stage III to signify locally unresectable disease and Stage IV to indicate metastatic disease.

INTRODUCTION

Cancers of the gallbladder are staged according to their depth of penetration and extent of spread. These cancers frequently spread to the liver, which is involved in 70% of patients at the time of surgical evaluation. Malignant tumors of the gallbladder can also directly invade other adjacent organs, particularly the common bile duct, the duodenum, and the transverse colon. Gallbladder cancers are insidious in their growth, often metastasizing early, before a diagnosis is made. Tumors can also perforate the wall of the gallbladder, eventually causing intra-abdominal metastases, carcinomatosis, and ascites. Because gallbladder cancer is uncommon and is usually diagnosed late, physicians have tended to ignore anatomic staging, even though its importance for survival, management, and prognosis has been emphasized. Many cases are not suspected clinically and first discovered at laparoscopy or incidentally by the pathologist. More than 75% of carcinomas of the gallbladder are associated with cholelithiasis. Survival correlates with the stage of disease.

ANATOMY

Primary Site. The gallbladder is a pear-shaped saccular organ located under the liver in the gallbladder fossa. It has three parts: a fundus, a body, and a neck that tapers into the cystic duct. The wall of the gallbladder is much thinner than that of the intestine and lacks a circular and transverse muscle layer. The wall has a mucosa (that is, an epithelial lining and lamina propria), a smooth muscle layer analogous to the muscularis propria of the small intestine, perimuscular connective tissue, and serosa. In contrast to the intestine, there is no submucosa. Along the attachment to the liver, no serosa exists, and the perimuscular connective tissue is continuous with the interlobular connective tissue of the liver. Tumors that arise in the cystic duct are classified according to the scheme for the extrahepatic bile ducts.

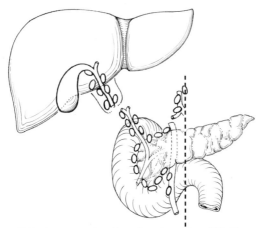

FIGURE 15.1. Regional lymph nodes of the gallbladder.

Regional Lymph Nodes. Accurate tumor staging requires that all lymph nodes that are removed be analyzed. Optimal histologic examination of a regional lymphadenectomy specimen should include analysis of a minimum of three lymph nodes. The regional lymph nodes include the following: hilar, celiac, periduodenal, peripancreatic, and superior mesenteric. The hilar nodes include the lymph nodes along the common bile duct, hepatic artery, portal vein, and cystic duct (Figure 15.1).

Metastatic Sites. Cancers of the gallbladder usually metastasize to the peritoneum and liver and occasionally to the lungs and pleura.

DEFINITIONS

Primary Tumor (T)

TX	Primary tumor cannot be assessed
T0	No evidence of primary tumor
Tis	Carcinoma *in situ*
T1	Tumor invades lamina propria or muscle layer
T1a	Tumor invades lamina propria (Figure 15.2)
T1b	Tumor invades muscle layer (Figure 15.2)
T2	Tumor invades perimuscular connective tissue; no extension beyond serosa or into liver (Figure 15.3)
T3	Tumor perforates the serosa (visceral peritoneum) and/or directly invades the liver and/or one other adjacent organ or structure, such as the stomach, duodenum, colon, pancreas, omentum, or extrahepatic bile ducts (Figures 15.4A, B)
T4	Tumor invades main portal vein or hepatic artery or invades two or more extrahepatic organs or structures (Figures 15.5A, B)

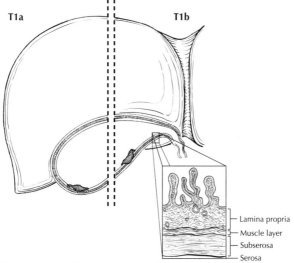

FIGURE 15.2. T1a is defined as tumor invading lamina propria; T1b is defined as tumor invading muscle layer.

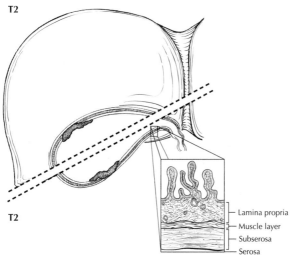

FIGURE 15.3. Two views of T2: tumor invading perimuscular connective tissue (illustration and inset below dotted line) and tumor with no extension beyond serosa into the liver (illustration above dotted line).

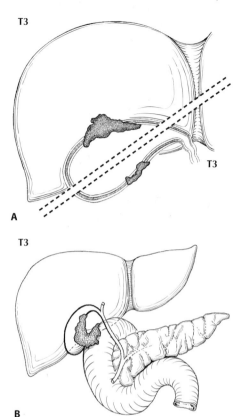

FIGURE 15.4. A. Two views of T3: tumor perforating the serosa (visceral peritoneum) (below the dotted line) and/or directly invading the liver (above the dotted line). **B.** T3 may also be defined as tumor invading one other adjacent organ or structure, such as the duodenum (as illustrated), or the stomach, colon, pancreas, omentum, or extrahepatic bile ducts.

Regional Lymph Nodes (N)

NX	Regional lymph nodes cannot be assessed
N0	No regional lymph node metastasis
N1	Regional lymph node metastasis (Figure 15.6)

Distant Metastasis (M)

MX	Distant metastasis cannot be assessed
M0	No distant metastasis
M1	Distant metastasis

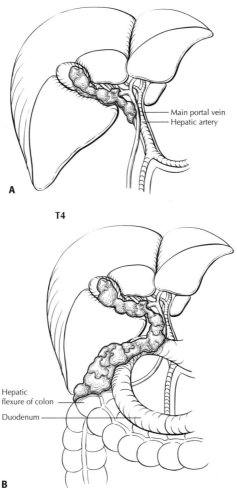

T4

Main portal vein
Hepatic artery

A

T4

Hepatic
flexure of colon
Duodenum

B

FIGURE 15.5. A. T4 is defined as tumor invading main portal vein or hepatic artery (as illustrated), or invading two or more extrahepatic organs or structures. **B.** T4 invading two or more extrahepatic organs or structures (here, colon and duodenum).

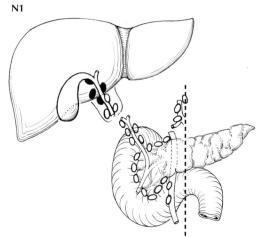

FIGURE 15.6. N1 is defined as metastasis to regional lymph nodes.

STAGE GROUPING

0	Tis	N0	M0
IA	T1	N0	M0
IB	T2	N0	M0
IIA	T3	N0	M0
IIB	T1	N1	M0
	T2	N1	M0
	T3	N1	M0
III	T4	Any N	M0
IV	Any T	Any N	M1

Extrahepatic Bile Ducts

(Sarcomas and carcinoid tumors are not included.)

| C24.0 | Extrahepatic bile duct | C24.8 | Overlapping lesion of the biliary tract | C24.9 | Biliary tract, NOS |

SUMMARY OF CHANGES

• The T and N classifications have been redefined and simplified.

• Invasion of the subepithelial fibro (muscular) connective tissue is classified as T1 irrespective of muscular invasion, which cannot always be noted because of the scarcity of muscle fibers in some bile duct segments.

• T2 is defined as invasion beyond the wall of the bile duct.

• The T classification allows one to separate locally invasive tumors into resectable (T3) and unresectable (T4).

• Invasion of branches of the portal vein (right or left), hepatic artery, or liver is classified as T3.

• Invasion of the main portal vein, common hepatic artery, and/or regional organs is classified as T4.

• The stage grouping has been changed to allow Stage III to signify locally unresectable disease and Stage IV to indicate metastatic disease.

INTRODUCTION

Malignant tumors can develop anywhere along the extrahepatic bile ducts (Figure 16.1). Of these tumors, 70–80% involve the confluence of the right and left hepatic ducts (hilar carcinomas), and about 20–30% arise more distally. Diffuse involvement of the ducts is rare, occurring in only about 2% of cases. All malignant tumors of the extrahepatic bile ducts inevitably cause partial or complete ductal obstruction. Because the bile ducts have a small diameter, the signs and symptoms of obstruction usually occur while tumors are relatively small. Because of their invasion of major vascular structures and direct extension to the liver, hilar carcinomas are more difficult to resect than those that arise distally and are associated with a worse prognosis (because of the low rate of resectability).

This TNM classification applies only to cancers arising in the extrahepatic bile ducts above the ampulla of Vater. This includes malignant tumors that develop in congenital choledochal cysts and tumors that arise in the intrapancreatic portion of the common bile duct. Patients with advanced (metastatic) disease and a primary tumor in the intrapancreatic portion of the common bile duct may be misclassified as having pancreatic cancer if surgical resection is not performed. In such cases, it is often impossible to determine (from radiographic images or endoscopy) whether a tumor arises from the intrapancreatic portion of the bile duct, the ampulla of Vater, or the pancreas. Tumors of the pancreas and ampulla of Vater are classified separately.

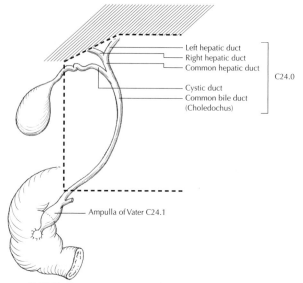

FIGURE 16.1. Anatomic sites of the extrahepatic bile ducts.

ANATOMY

Primary Site. Emerging from the transverse scissura of the liver are the right and left hepatic bile ducts, which join to form the common hepatic duct. The cystic duct, which connects to the gallbladder, joins the common hepatic duct to form the common bile duct, which passes posterior to the first part of the duodenum, traverses the head of the pancreas, and then enters the second part of the duodenum through the ampulla of Vater. Histologically, the bile ducts are lined by a single layer of tall, uniform columnar cells. The mucosa usually forms irregular pleats or small longitudinal folds. The walls of the bile ducts have a layer of subepithelial connective tissue and muscle fibers. It should be noted that the muscle fibers are most prominent in the distal segment of the common bile duct. More proximally, the muscle fibers are sparse or absent, and the walls of the bile ducts consist largely of fibrous tissue.

Regional Lymph Nodes. Accurate tumor staging requires that all lymph nodes that are removed be analyzed. Optimal histologic examination of a regional lymphadenectomy specimen should include analysis of a minimum of three lymph nodes. The regional lymph nodes are the same as those listed for gallbladder cancer and include the following: hilar, celiac, periduodenal, peripancreatic, and superior mesenteric. The hilar nodes include the lymph nodes along the common bile duct, hepatic artery, portal vein, and cystic duct.

Metastatic Sites. Extrahepatic bile duct carcinomas can extend to the liver, pancreas, ampulla of Vater, duodenum, colon, omentum, stomach, or gallbladder. Tumors arising in the right or left hepatic ducts usually extend proximally

FIGURE 16.2. Two views of T1: both tumors are confined to the bile duct histologically.

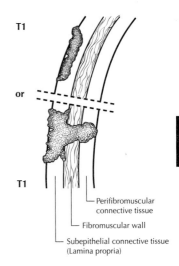

T1

or

T1

└ Perifibromuscular connective tissue

└ Fibromuscular wall

└ Subepithelial connective tissue (Lamina propria)

into the liver or distally to the common hepatic duct. Neoplasms from the cystic duct invade the gallbladder, common bile duct, or both. Carcinomas that arise in the distal segment of the common bile duct can spread to the pancreas, duodenum, stomach, colon, or omentum. Distant metastases usually occur late in the course of the disease and are most often found in the liver, lungs, and peritoneum.

DEFINITIONS

Primary Tumor (T)

TX   Primary tumor cannot be assessed

T0   No evidence of primary tumor

Tis   Carcinoma *in situ*

T1   Tumor confined to the bile duct histologically (Figure 16.2)

T2   Tumor invades beyond the wall of the bile duct (Figure 16.3)

T2

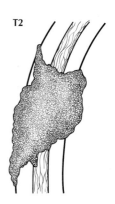

FIGURE 16.3. T2 is defined as tumor that invades beyond the wall of the bile duct.

T3   Tumor invades the liver, gallbladder, pancreas, and/or ipsilateral branches of the portal vein (right or left) or hepatic artery (right or left) (Figures 16.4A–C)

T4   Tumor invades any of the following: main portal vein or its branches bilaterally, common hepatic artery, or other adjacent structures, such as the colon, stomach, duodenum, or abdominal wall (Figures 16.5A, B)

Regional Lymph Nodes (N)

NX   Regional lymph nodes cannot be assessed
N0   No regional lymph node metastasis
N1   Regional lymph node metastasis

Distant Metastasis (M)

MX   Distant metastasis cannot be assessed
M0   No distant metastasis
M1   Distant metastasis

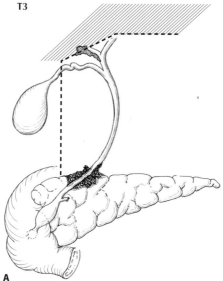

A

FIGURE 16.4. A. T3 is defined as tumor invading the liver (as illustrated), gallbladder, pancreas, and/or ipsilateral branches of the portal vein (right or left) or hepatic artery (right or left).

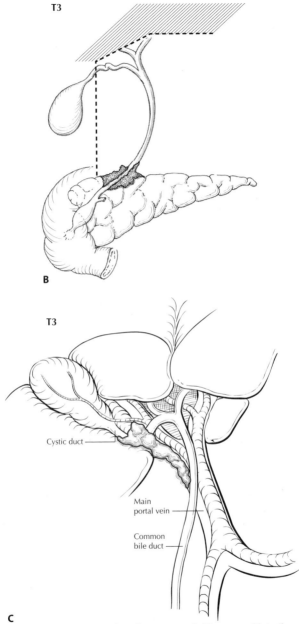

FIGURE 16.4. B. T3 tumor invading the pancreas. **C.** T3 tumor with ipsilateral invasion of the right portal vein and gallbladder.

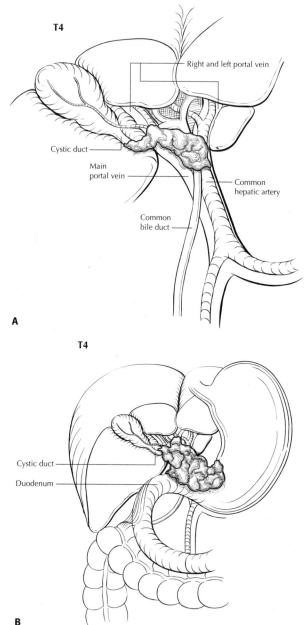

FIGURE 16.5. A. T4 is defined as tumor that invades any of the following: main portal vein or its branches bilaterally, common hepatic artery, or other adjacent structures, such as the colon, stomach, duodenum, or abdominal wall. Here, tumor invades the common hepatic artery and bilateral branches of the portal vein. **B.** T4 tumor invading the stomach.

STAGE GROUPING

0	Tis	N0	M0
IA	T1	N0	M0
IB	T2	N0	M0
IIA	T3	N0	M0
IIB	T1	N1	M0
	T2	N1	M0
	T3	N1	M0
III	T4	Any N	M0
IV	Any T	Any N	M1

16

Ampulla of Vater

(Carcinoid tumors and other neuroendocrine tumors are not included.)

C24.1   Ampulla of Vater

SUMMARY OF CHANGES

- There is no longer a distinction between T3 and T4 on the basis of the depth of pancreatic invasion.
- The stage grouping has been revised.
- Stage I has been replaced with Stage IA and Stage IB.
- Stage II has been replaced with Stage IIA and Stage IIB.
- Node positive disease has been moved to Stage IIB to retain consistency with the staging of tumors of the bile duct and of the pancreas.

INTRODUCTION

The ampulla of Vater is strategically located at the confluence of the pancreatic and common bile ducts. Most tumors that arise in this small structure obstruct the common bile duct, causing jaundice, abdominal pain, and occasionally pancreatitis. Clinically and pathologically, carcinomas of the ampulla may be difficult to differentiate from those arising in the head of the pancreas or in the distal segment of the common bile duct. Primary cancers of the ampulla are not common, although they constitute a high proportion of the malignant tumors occurring in the duodenum. Tumors of the ampulla must be differentiated from those arising in the second part of the duodenum and invading the ampulla, which are staged as small bowel tumors. Carcinomas of the ampulla and peri-ampullary region are often associated with the familial adenomatous polyposis syndrome.

ANATOMY

Primary Site. The ampulla is a small dilated duct less than 1.5 cm long, formed in most individuals by the union of the terminal segments of the pancreatic and common bile ducts (Figure 17.1). In 42% of individuals, however, the ampulla is the termination of the common duct only, the pancreatic duct having its own entrance into the duodenum adjacent to ampulla. In these individuals, the ampulla may be difficult to locate or even nonexistent. The ampulla opens into the duodenum, usually on the posterior-medial wall, through a small mucosal elevation, the duodenal papilla, which is also called the ampulla of Vater. Although carcinomas can arise in the mucosa of either the lining of the ampulla or the duodenal surface of the duodenal papilla, they most commonly arise near the junction of the two types of mucosa at the ampullary orifice. Nearly all cancers that arise in this area are well-differentiated adenocarcinomas. They have a variety of designations, including carcinoma of the ampulla of Vater, carci-

---

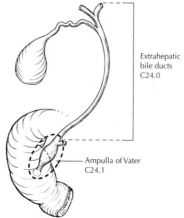

FIGURE 17.1. Anatomic site of the ampulla of Vater.

noma of the periampullary portion of the duodenum, and carcinoma of the peripapillary portion of the duodenum. It may not be possible to determine the exact site of origin for large tumors.

Regional Lymph Nodes. A rich lymphatic network surrounds the pancreas and periampullary region, and accurate tumor staging requires that all lymph nodes that are removed by analyzed. Optimal histologic examination of a pancreaticoduodenectomy specimen should include analysis of a minimum of 10 lymph nodes. The regional lymph nodes are the peripancreatic lymph nodes, which also include the lymph nodes along the hepatic artery, celiac axis, and pyloric regions (Figures 17.2, 17.3). Anatomic division of regional lymph nodes is not necessary; however, separately submitted lymph nodes should be reported as submitted.

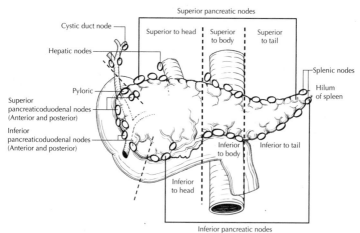

FIGURE 17.2. Regional lymph nodes of the ampulla of Vater.

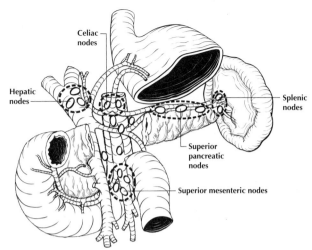

FIGURE 17.3. Regional lymph nodes to the ampulla of Vater, namely the proximal mesenteric and common bile duct nodes. View shows the pancreatic body cut away to reveal the proximal mesenteric lymph nodes.

Metastatic Sites. Tumors of the ampulla may infiltrate adjacent structures, such as the wall of the duodenum, the head of the pancreas, and extrahepatic bile ducts. Metastatic disease is most commonly found in the liver and peritoneum and is less commonly seen in the lungs and pleura.

DEFINITIONS

Primary Tumor (T)

TX Primary tumor cannot be assessed
T0 No evidence of primary tumor
Tis Carcinoma *in situ*
T1 Tumor limited to ampulla of Vater or sphincter of Oddi (Figure 17.4)
T2 Tumor invades duodenal wall (Figure 17.5)
T3 Tumor invades pancreas (Figure 17.6)
T4 Tumor invades peripancreatic soft tissues or other adjacent organs or structures (Figure 17.7)

Regional Lymph Nodes (N)

NX Regional lymph nodes cannot be assessed
N0 No regional lymph node metastasis
N1 Regional lymph node metastasis (Figures 17.8A–C for tumors located in the head of the pancreas)

Distant Metastasis (M)

MX Distant metastasis cannot be assessed
M0 No distant metastasis
M1 Distant metastasis (Figures 17.9A, B)

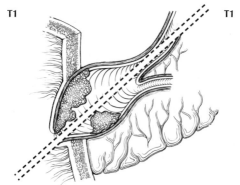

FIGURE 17.4. Two views of T1: tumor limited to ampulla of Vater (below dotted line) or sphincter of Oddi (tumor shown above dotted line).

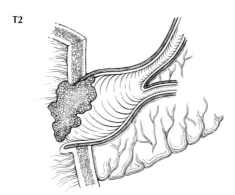

FIGURE 17.5. T2 tumor invading duodenal wall.

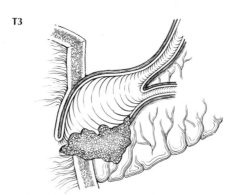

FIGURE 17.6. T3 tumor invading pancreas.

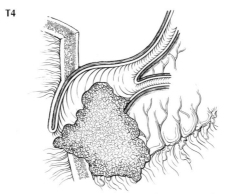

FIGURE 17.7. T4 tumor invading peripancreatic soft tissues or other adjacent organs or structures.

17

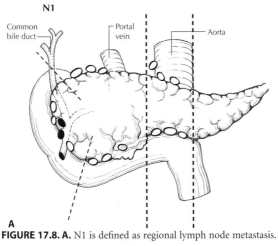

A
FIGURE 17.8. A. N1 is defined as regional lymph node metastasis.

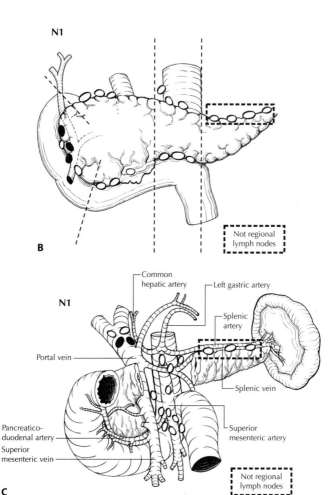

FIGURE 17.8. B, C. N1 is defined as regional lymph node metastasis.

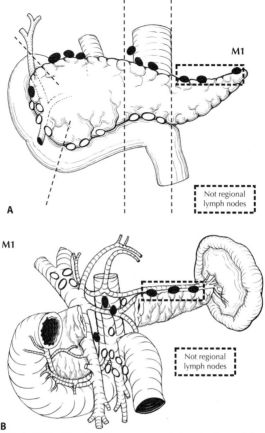

FIGURE 17.9. A. M1 is defined as distant metastasis, here to those of the tail of the pancreas. **B.** M1 is defined as distant metastasis, here to the splenic lymph nodes.

STAGE GROUPING

0	Tis	N0	M0
IA	T1	N0	M0
IB	T2	N0	M0
IIA	T3	N0	M0
IIB	T1	N1	M0
	T2	N1	M0
	T3	N1	M0
III	T4	Any N	M0
IV	Any T	Any N	M1

Exocrine Pancreas

(Endocrine tumors arising from the islets of Langerhans and carcinoid tumors are not included.)

C25.0	Head of pancreas	C25.3	Pancreatic duct	C25.8	Overlapping lesion of
C25.1	Body of pancreas	C25.7	Other specified parts		pancreas
C25.2	Tail of pancreas		of pancreas	C25.9	Pancreas, NOS

SUMMARY OF CHANGES

- The T classification reflects the distinction between potentially resectable (T3) and locally advanced (T4) primary pancreatic tumors.

- Stage grouping has been changed to allow Stage III to signify unresectable, locally advanced pancreatic cancer, while Stage IV is reserved for patients with metastatic disease.

INTRODUCTION

In the United States, pancreatic cancer is the second most common tumor of the gastrointestinal tract and the fifth leading cause of cancer-related death in adults. The disease is difficult to diagnose, especially in its early stages. Most pancreatic cancers arise in the head of the pancreas, often causing bile duct obstruction that results in clinically evident jaundice. Cancers that arise in either the body or the tail of the pancreas are insidious in their development and often far advanced when first detected. Most pancreatic cancers are adenocarcinomas, which usually originate from the pancreatic duct cells. Surgical resection remains the only potentially curative approach, although multimodality therapy that includes innovative systemic agents and often radiation therapy is available.

Staging of exocrine pancreas cancers depends on the size and extent of the primary tumor. This TNM classification does not apply to endocrine tumors.

ANATOMY

Primary Site. The pancreas is a long, coarsely lobulated gland that lies transversely across the posterior abdomen and extends from the duodenum to the splenic hilum. The organ is divided into a head with a small uncinate process, a neck, a body, and a tail. The anatomic subsites of the pancreas are illustrated in Figure 18.1. The anterior aspect of the body of the pancreas is in direct contact with the posterior wall of the stomach; posteriorly, the pancreas extends to the aorta, splenic vein, and left kidney.

Tumors on the head of the pancreas are those arising to the right of the superior mesenteric-portal vein confluence (Figure 18.2, posterior view of pancreatic head). The uncinate process is part of the pancreatic head. Tumors of the body of the pancreas are roughly defined as those arising between the superior mesenteric-portal vein confluence and the aorta. Tumors of the tail of the pancreas are those arising between the aorta and the hilum of the spleen.

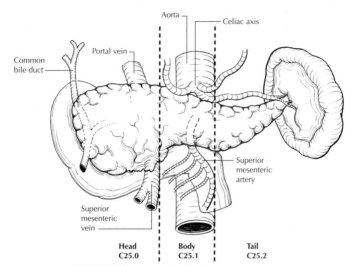

FIGURE 18.1. Anatomic subsites of the pancreas.

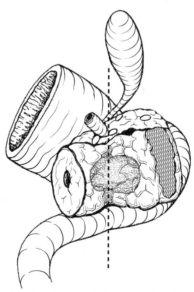

FIGURE 18.2. Posterior view of pancreatic head with dotted line indicating the location of the confluence of the portal and superior mesenteric veins. The hatched area shows the uncinate process margin.

Regional Lymph Nodes. A rich lymphatic network surrounds the pancreas and accurate tumor staging requires that all lymph nodes that are removed be analyzed. Optimal histologic examination of a pancreaticoduodenectomy specimen should include analysis of a minimum of 10 lymph nodes, although pathologic analysis of fewer than 10 lymph nodes may still result in a pN0 designation. The nomenclature for the regional lymph nodes of the pancreas is not standardized, but the main classification systems currently in use are descriptive and based on the anatomic location of the nodes. Accordingly, the pancreas has two broad groups of regional nodes: those that form a ring around the organ and those surrounding the adjacent large vessels (the abdominal aorta and its major branches including the celiac axis, the superior mesenteric artery, and the renal arteries). The specific nodal groups include: the anterior pancreaticoduodenal nodes (superior and inferior), the posterior pancreaticoduodenal nodes (superior and inferior), the pyloric nodes (adjacent to the pylorus), the gastroduodenal nodes (adjacent to the gastroduodenal artery), the hepatic nodes (adjacent to the common bile duct and the hepatic artery), the cystic node (adjacent to the choledochal cystic duct), the superior mesenteric nodes, the celiac nodes, the supra- and infrapancreatic nodes (located along the superior and inferior borders of the pancreas, respectively), the mesocolic nodes, the splenic nodes, and the gastrosplenic nodes. Some anatomic studies have shown primary lymphatic drainage into the renal nodes as well. Although the nodes located closest to the regional subdivisions of the pancreas (head, body, and tail) are the primary lymphatic drainage stations for those zones, all of the specific nodal groups named above are included in the N category for the pancreas (Figures 18.3, 18.4). Anatomic division of the regional lymph nodes is not necessary; however, separately submitted lymph nodes should be reported as submitted.

Metastatic Sites. Distant spread occurs commonly to the liver, peritoneal cavity, and lungs. Metastases to other sites are uncommon (or rarely detected),

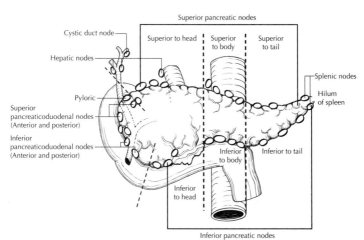

FIGURE 18.3. Regional lymph nodes of the pancreas (anterior view).

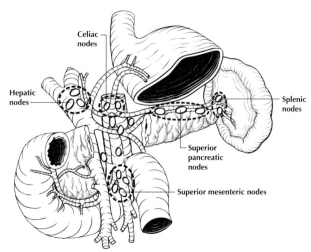

FIGURE 18.4. Regional lymph nodes of the pancreas (anterior view with pancreatic body removed to reveal retroperitoneal vessels and lymph nodes).

possibly because of the short interval from diagnosis of distant metastasis to death.

DEFINITIONS

Primary Tumor (T)

TX Primary tumor cannot be assessed
T0 No evidence of primary tumor
Tis Carcinoma *in situ*
T1 Tumor limited to the pancreas 2 cm or less in greatest dimension (Figure 18.5)
T2 Tumor limited to the pancreas more than 2 cm in greatest dimension (Figure 18.5)
T3 Tumor extends beyond the pancreas but without involvement of the celiac axis or the superior mesenteric artery (Figures 18.6A–C)
T4 Tumor involves the celiac axis or the superior mesenteric artery (unresectable primary tumor) (Figure 18.7)

Regional Lymph Nodes (N)

NX Regional lymph nodes cannot be assessed
N0 No regional lymph node metastasis
N1 Regional lymph node metastasis (Figures 18.8A–D)

Distant Metastasis (M)

MX Distant metastasis cannot be assessed
M0 No distant metastasis
M1 Distant metastasis

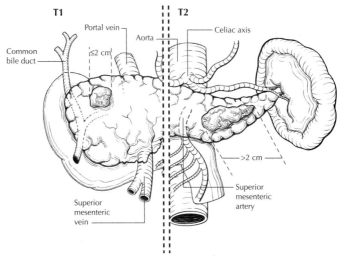

FIGURE 18.5. T1 (left of dotted line) is defined as tumor limited to the pancreas 2 cm or less in greatest dimension. T2 (right of dotted line) is defined as tumor limited to the pancreas more than 2 cm in greatest dimension.

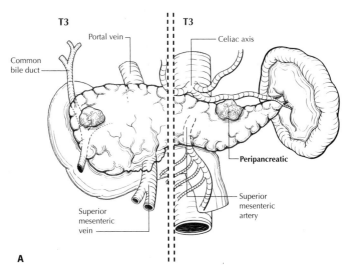

A

FIGURE 18.6. A. Two views of T3, which is defined as tumor that extends beyond the pancreas but without involvement of the celiac axis or the superior mesenteric artery. Left of the dotted line: tumor invades the common bile duct without involving the superior mesenteric artery. Right of the dotted line: tumor invades peripancreatic tissues without involving the celiac axis.

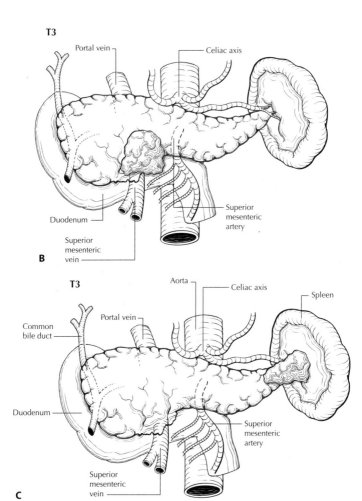

FIGURE 18.6. B. T3: tumor invades duodenum without involvement of the superior mesenteric artery. **C.** T3: tumor invades spleen without involvement of celiac axis or superior mesenteric artery.

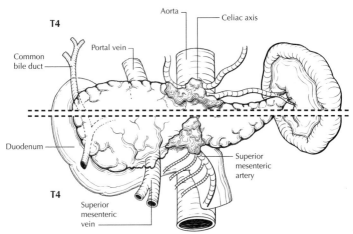

FIGURE 18.7. Two views of T4, which is defined as tumor involving the celiac axis (above dotted line) or (below dotted line) the superior mesenteric artery (unresectable primary tumor).

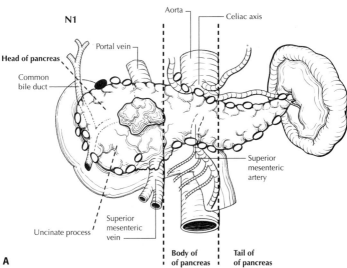

A

FIGURE 18.8. A. N1 is defined as regional lymph node metastasis. Here, the primary tumor and single nodal metastasis are located within the head of pancreas.

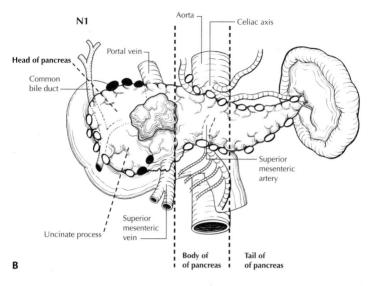

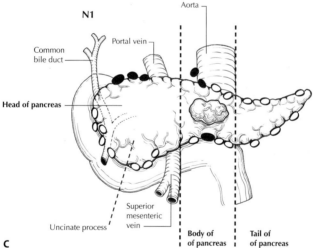

FIGURE 18.8. N1 is defined as regional lymph node metastasis. **B.** Here, the primary tumor and multiple nodal metastases are located in the head of pancreas. **C.** Here, the primary tumor is located in the body of pancreas with multiple nodal metastases in the head and body of pancreas.

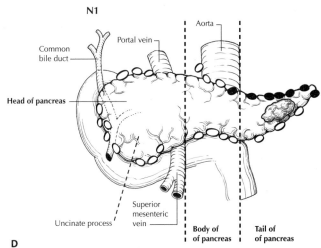

D

FIGURE 18.8. D. N1 is defined as regional lymph node metastasis. Here, the primary tumor is located in the tail of pancreas with multiple nodal metastases in the tail of pancreas and hilum of spleen.

STAGE GROUPING

0	Tis	N0	M0
IA	T1	N0	M0
IB	T2	N0	M0
IIA	T3	N0	M0
IIB	T1	N1	M0
	T2	N1	M0
	T3	N1	M0
III	T4	Any N	M0
IV	Any T	Any N	M1

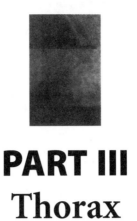

PART III
Thorax

Lung

(Sarcomas and other rare tumors are not included.)

C34.0	Main bronchus	C34.3	Lower lobe, lung	C34.9	Lung, NOS
C34.1	Upper lobe, lung	C34.8	Overlapping lesion of		
C34.2	Middle lobe, lung		lung		

SUMMARY OF CHANGES

• The definitions of TNM and the Stage Grouping for this chapter have not changed from the Fifth Edition.

INTRODUCTION

Lung cancer is among the most common malignancies in the Western world and is the leading cause of cancer deaths in both men and women. It is one of the few tumors with a known carcinogen, namely tobacco, contributing to its etiology. In recent years we have come to appreciate that the initiation of lung cancer is a complex process that also involves certain biologic factors, such as the body's ability to process carcinogens. This disease is usually not diagnosed early, and therefore the overall 5-year survival rate is approximately 15%. The treatment of lung cancer depends on the extent of disease, the location of the primary tumor, and the presence or absence of medical comorbidities. The assessment of extrapulmonary intrathoracic and extrathoracic metastasis is important for staging and patient evaluation.

ANATOMY

Primary Site. Carcinomas of the lung arise either from the alveolar lining cells of the pulmonary parenchyma or from the mucosa of the tracheobronchial tree. The trachea, which lies in the middle mediastinum, divides into the right and left main bronchi, which extend into the right and left lungs, respectively. The bronchi then subdivide into the lobar bronchi for the upper, middle, and lower lobes on the right and the upper and lower lobes on the left. The lungs are encased in membranes called the visceral pleura. The inside of the chest cavity is lined by a similar membrane called the parietal pleura. The potential space between these two membranes is called the pleural space. The mediastinum contains the heart, thymus, great vessels, and other structures between the lungs.

The great vessels include:

Aorta
Superior vena cava
Inferior vena cava
Main pulmonary artery
Intrapericardial segments of the trunk of the right and left pulmonary artery
Intrapericardial segments of the superior and inferior right and left pulmonary
    veins

The main anatomical subsites are shown in Figure 19.1:

C34.0: Main bronchus
C34.1: Upper lobe
C34.2: Middle lobe
C34.3: Lower lobe

Regional Lymph Nodes. All regional lymph nodes are above the diaphragm. They include the intrathoracic, scalene, and supraclavicular nodes. For purposes of staging, the intrathoracic nodes include the following:

Mediastinal:
Paratracheal (including those that may be designated tracheobronchial—that is, lower paratracheal, including azygous)
Pre- and retrotracheal (includes precarinal)
Aortic (includes aortopulmonary window, periaortic, ascending aortic, and phrenic)
Subcarinal
Periesophageal
Inferior pulmonary ligament

Intrapulmonary:
Hilar (proximal lobar)
Peribronchial
Intrapulmonary (includes interlobar, lobar, and segmental)

Figure 19.2 illustrates lymph node maps of the lungs. All N1 nodes lie distal to the mediastinal pleural reflection and *within the visceral pleura*. All N2 nodes lie within the mediastinal pleural envelope on the ipsilateral side.

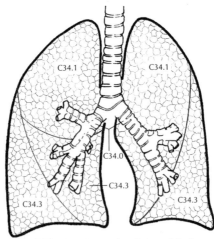

FIGURE 19.1. Anatomic subsites of the lung.

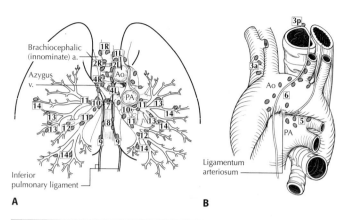

N2 nodes:		N1 nodes:
1 Highest medistinal	5 Subaortic	10 Hilar
2 Upper paratracheal	6 Para-aortic	11 Interlobar
3 Prevascular and retrotracheal	7 Subcarinal	12 Lobar nodes bronchi
4 Lower paratracheal	8 Paraesophageal	13 Segmental
	9 Pulmonary ligament	14 Subsegmental

FIGURE 19.2. Lymph node maps of the lung.

Distant Metastatic Sites. The most common metastatic sites are the brain, bones, adrenal glands, contralateral lung, liver, pericardium, and kidneys. However, virtually any organ can be a site of metastases.

DEFINITIONS OF TNM

Primary Tumor (T)

TX Primary tumor cannot be assessed, or tumor proven by the presence of malignant cells in sputum or bronchial washings but not visualized by imaging or bronchoscopy

T0 No evidence of primary tumor

Tis Carcinoma *in situ*

T1 Tumor 3 cm or less in greatest dimension, surrounded by lung or visceral pleura, without bronchoscopic evidence of invasion more proximal than the lobar bronchus[1] (i.e., not in the main bronchus) (Figure 19.3)

T2 Tumor with any of the following features of size or extent (Figure 19.4):
  • More than 3 cm in greatest dimension
  • Involves main bronchus, 2 cm or more distal to the carina
  • Invades the visceral pleura
  • Associated with atelectasis or obstructive pneumonitis that extends to the hilar region but does not involve the entire lung

T3 Tumor of any size that directly invades any of the following: chest wall (including superior sulcus tumors), diaphragm, mediastinal pleura, parietal pericardium; or tumor in the main bronchus less than 2 cm distal to

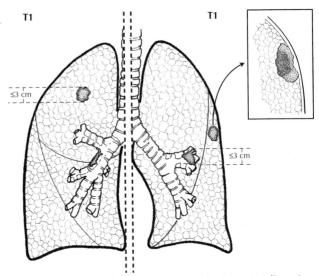

FIGURE 19.3. Two views of T1 showing tumor 3 cm or less in greatest dimension.

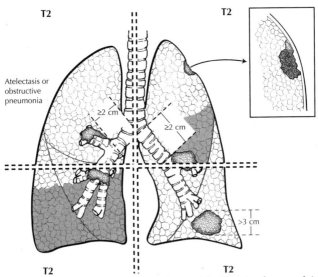

FIGURE 19.4. T2 is defined as a tumor with any of the following features of size or extent: more than 3 cm in greatest dimension; involving main bronchus, 2 cm or more distal to the carina; invades the visceral pleura; associated with atelectasis or obstructive pneumonitis that extends to the hilar region but does not involve the entire lung.

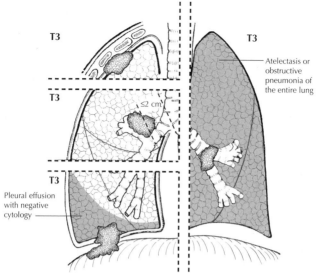

FIGURE 19.5. T3 is defined as a tumor of any size that directly invades any of the following: chest wall (including superior sulcus tumors), diaphragm, mediastinal pleura, parietal pericardium; or tumor in the main bronchus less than 2 cm distal to the carina, but without involvement of the carina; or associated atelectasis or obstructive pneumonitis of the entire lung.

the carina, but without involvement of the carina; or associated atelectasis or obstructive pneumonitis of the entire lung (Figure 19.5)

T4   Tumor of any size that invades any of the following: mediastinum, heart, great vessels, trachea, esophagus, vertebral body, carina; or separate tumor nodules in the same lobe; or tumor with malignant pleural effusion[2] (Figures 19.6A–E)

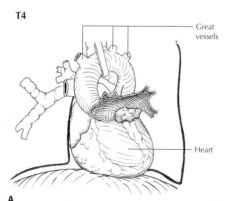

A
FIGURE 19.6. A. Tumor invasion of the heart and great vessels.

T4

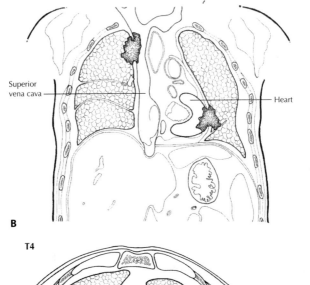

Superior
vena cava

Heart

B

T4

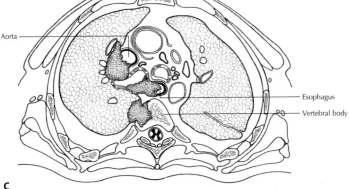

Aorta

Esophagus

Vertebral body

C

FIGURE 19.6. B. Tumor invasion of the superior vena cava and heart. **C.** Tumor invasion of the aorta, esophagus, and vertebral body.

Regional Lymph Nodes (N)

NX Regional lymph nodes cannot be assessed

N0 No regional lymph node metastasis

N1 Metastasis to ipsilateral peribronchial and/or ipsilateral hilar lymph nodes, and intrapulmonary nodes including involvement by direct extension of the primary tumor (Figure 19.7)

N2 Metastasis to ipsilateral mediastinal and/or subcarinal lymph nodes(s) (Figure 19.8)

N3 Metastasis to contralateral mediastinal, contralateral hilar, ipsilateral or contralateral scalene, or supraclavicular lymph node(s) (Figure 19.9)

Distant Metastasis (M)

MX   Distant metastasis cannot be assessed
M0   No distant metastasis
M1   Distant metastasis present[3] (Figure 19.9)

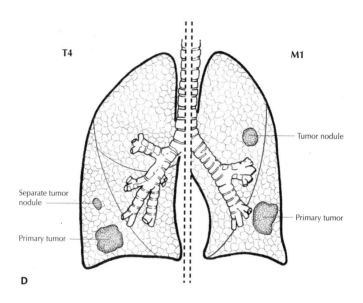

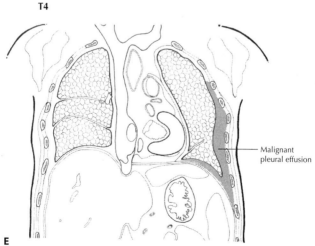

FIGURE 19.6. D. N1 is defined as a separate tumor nodule(s) in the same lobe. M1 is defined as a separate tumor nodule(s) in a different lobe (ipsilateral or contralateral). **E.** Tumor with malignant pleural effusion (see note 2).

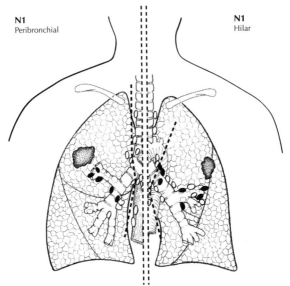

FIGURE 19.7. N1 is defined as metastasis to ipsilateral peribronchial (left side of diagram) and/or ipsilateral hilar lymph nodes (right side of diagram), and intrapulmonary nodes including involvement by direct extension of the primary tumor.

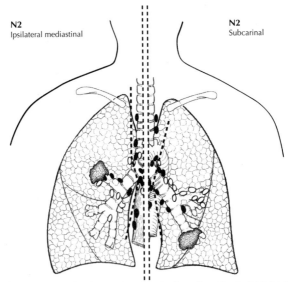

FIGURE 19.8. N2 is defined as metastasis to ipsilateral mediastinal (right side of diagram) and/or subcarinal lymph nodes(s) (left side of diagram).

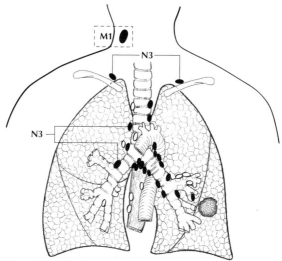

FIGURE 19.9. N3 is defined as metastasis to contralateral mediastinal, contralateral hilar, ipsilateral or contralateral scalene, or supraclavicular lymph node(s) whereas M1 is defined as distant metastasis.

STAGE GROUPING

Occult carcinoma	TX	N0	M0
0	Tis	N0	M0
IA	T1	N0	M0
IB	T2	N0	M0
IIA	T1	N1	M0
IIB	T2	N1	M0
	T3	N0	M0
IIIA	T1	N2	M0
	T2	N2	M0
	T3	N1	M0
	T3	N2	M0
IIIB	Any T	N3	M0
	T4	Any N	M0
IV	Any T	Any N	M1

NOTES

1. The uncommon superficial tumor of any size with its invasive component limited to the bronchial wall, which may extend proximal to the main bronchus, is also classified T1.
2. Most pleural effusions associated with lung cancer are due to tumor. However, there are a few patients in whom multiple cytopathologic examinations of pleural fluid are negative for tumor. In these cases, fluid is non-bloody and is not an

exudate. Such patients may be further evaluated by videothoracoscopy (VATS) and direct pleural biopsies. When these elements and clinical judgment dictate that the effusion is not related to the tumor, the effusion should be excluded as a staging element and the patient should be staged T1, T2, or T3.

3. M1 includes separate tumor nodule(s) in a different lobe (ipsilateral or contralateral).

Pleural Mesothelioma

(Tumors metastatic to the pleura and lung tumors that have extended to the pleural surfaces are not included.)

C38.4   Pleura NOS

SUMMARY OF CHANGES

- The AJCC has adopted the staging system proposed by the International Mesothelioma Working Group (IMIG) in 1995. It is based on updated information about the relationships between tumor (T) and N status and overall survival. This staging system applies only to tumors arising in the pleura.

- T categories have been redefined

- T1 lesions have been divided into T1a and T1b, leading to the division of Stage I into Stage IA and Stage IB.

- T3 is defined as locally advanced but potentially resectable tumor.

- T4 is defined as locally advanced, technically unresectable tumor.

- Stage II no longer involves tumors with nodal metastasis; all nodal metastasis is categorized in Stage III or Stage IV.

INTRODUCTION

Malignant mesotheliomas are relatively rare tumors that arise from the mesothelium lining the pleural, pericardial, and peritoneal cavities. They represent less than 2% of all malignant tumors. The most common risk factor for malignant mesotheliomas is previous exposure to asbestos. The latency period between asbestos exposure and the development of malignant mesothelioma is generally 20 years or more. Although peritoneal mesotheliomas are thought to occur in individuals who have had heavier exposure than those with pleural mesothelioma, there is no clearly documented relationship between the amount of asbestos exposure and the subsequent development of this neoplasm. Malignant mesotheliomas were previously thought to be virulent tumors. However, this impression was probably related to the fact that most mesotheliomas are diagnosed when they are already at an advanced stage. Recent data indicate that the clinical and biological behavior of mesotheliomas is variable and that most mesotheliomas grow relatively slowly.

All mesotheliomas are fundamentally epithelial tumors. However, their morphology ranges from a pure epithelial appearance to an entirely sarcomatoid or even desmoplastic appearance. Distinguishing the pleiomorphic histology of mesotheliomas from that of other neoplasms can be difficult, especially for the pure epithelial mesotheliomas, which may closely resemble metastatic adenocarcinoma. Therefore, confirmation of the histologic diagnosis by immunohistochemistry and/or electron microscopy is essential.

During the past 30 years, many staging systems have been proposed for malignant pleural mesothelioma. The first staging system for this disease

---

published by the American Joint Committee on Cancer (AJCC), and simultaneously accepted by the International Union Against Cancer, appeared in the fifth edition of the AJCC Cancer Staging Manual. The staging system described here represents adoption of the one proposed in 1995 by the International Mesothelioma Interest Group (IMIG), which is based on updated information about the relationships between tumor (T) and N status and overall survival. Although this system has been validated by several surgical reports, it will probably require revision in the future as further data in larger numbers of patients become available. This staging system applies only to tumors arising in the pleura. Peritoneal and pericardial mesotheliomas are rare and do not lend themselves easily to a TNM staging system.

ANATOMY

Primary Site. The mesothelium covers the external surface of the lungs and the inside of the chest wall. It is usually composed of flat, tightly connected cells no more than one layer thick.

Regional Lymph Nodes. The regional lymph nodes include internal mammary, intrathoracic, scalene, and supraclavicular. The regional lymph node map and nomenclature adopted for the mesothelioma staging system is identical to that used for lung cancer. See Chapter 19 and Figure 19.2 for a detailed list and diagram of intrathoracic lymph nodes. For pN, histologic examination of a mediastinal lymphadenectomy or lymph node sampling specimen will ordinarily include regional nodes taken from the ipsilateral N1 and N2 nodal stations. Contralateral and supraclavicular nodes may be available if a mediastinoscopy or node biopsy is also performed.

Distant Metastatic Sites. Advanced malignant pleural mesotheliomas often metastasize widely to uncommon sites, including retroperitoneal lymph nodes, the brain and spine, or even organs such as the thyroid or prostate. However, the most frequent sites of metastatic disease are the peritoneum, contralateral pleura, and lung.

DEFINITIONS OF TNM

IMIG Staging System for Diffuse Malignant Pleural Mesothelioma

Primary Tumor (T)

TX   Primary tumor cannot be assessed

T0   No evidence of primary tumor

T1   Tumor involves ipsilateral parietal pleura, with or without focal involvement of visceral pleura

T1a   Tumor involves ipsilateral parietal (mediastinal, diaphragmatic) pleura; no involvement of the visceral pleura (Figure 20.1)

T1b   Tumor involves ipsilateral parietal (mediastinal, diaphragmatic) pleura, with focal involvement of the visceral pleura (Figure 20.1)

T2   Tumor involves any of the ipsilateral pleural surfaces with at least one of the following (Figure 20.2):

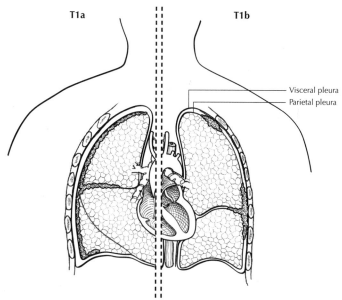

FIGURE 20.1. T1a (left) shows no involvement of the visceral pleura. T1b (right) involves ipsilateral parietal pleura, with focal involvement of the visceral pleura.

20

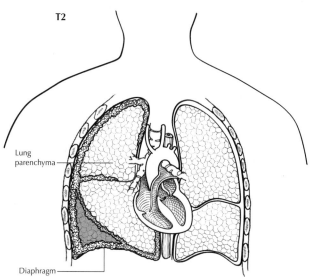

FIGURE 20.2. T2 involves any of the ipsilateral pleural surfaces with at least one of the following: confluent visceral pleural tumor (including fissure); invasion of diaphragmatic muscle (as illustrated); and/or invasion of lung parenchyma (as illustrated).

- Confluent visceral pleural tumor (including fissure)
- Invasion of diaphragmatic muscle
- Invasion of lung parenchyma

T3[1]   Tumor involves any of the ipsilateral pleural surfaces, with at least one of the following (Figure 20.3):
- Invasion of the endothoracic fascia
- Invasion into mediastinal fat
- Solitary focus of tumor invading the soft tissues of the chest wall
- Non-transmural involvement of the pericardium

T4[2]   Tumor involves any of the ipsilateral pleural surfaces, with at least one of the following (Figure 20.4):
- Diffuse or multifocal invasion of soft tissues of the chest wall
- Any involvement of rib
- Invasion through the diaphragm to the peritoneum
- Invasion of any mediastinal organ(s)
- Direct extension to the contralateral pleura
- Invasion into the spine
- Extension to the internal surface of the pericardium
- Pericardial effusion with positive cytology
- Invasion of the myocardium
- Invasion of the brachial plexus

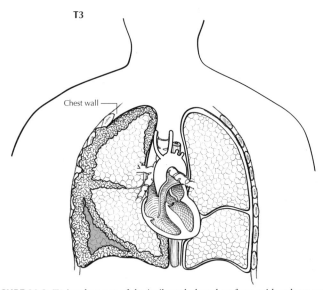

FIGURE 20.3. T3 involves any of the ipsilateral pleural surfaces, with at least one of the following: invasion of the endothoracic fascia; invasion into mediastinal fat; solitary focus of tumor invading the soft tissues of the chest wall (as illustrated); and/or non-transmural involvement of the pericardium.

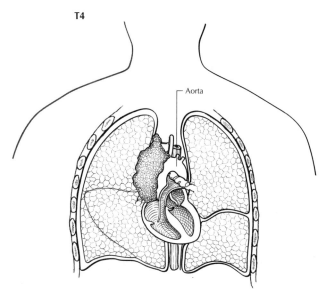

T4

— Aorta

FIGURE 20.4. T4 involves any of the ipsilateral pleural surfaces with at least one additional parameter, such as extension to the internal surface of the pericardium as illustrated here. (The full list of additional parameters is provided under Definitions of TNM.)

20

Regional Lymph Nodes (N)

NX   Regional lymph nodes cannot be assessed
N0   No regional lymph node metastases
N1   Metastases in the ipsilateral bronchopulmonary and/or hilar lymph node(s)
N2   Metastases in the subcarinal lymph node(s) and/or the ipsilateral internal mammary or mediastinal lymph node(s)
N3   Metastases in the contralateral mediastinal, internal mammary, or hilar lymph node(s), and/or the ipsilateral or contralateral supraclavicular or scalene lymph node(s)

Distant Metastasis (M)

MX   Distant metastasis cannot be assessed
M0   No distant metastasis
M1   Distant metastasis

STAGE GROUPING

I	T1	N0	M0
IA	T1a	N0	M0
IB	T1b	N0	M0
II	T2	N0	M0

III	T1, T2	N1	M0
	T1, T2	N2	M0
	T3	N0, N1, N2	M0
IV	T4	Any N	M0
	Any T	N3	M0
	Any T	Any N	M1

NOTES

1. T3 describes locally advanced but potentially resectable tumor.
2. T4 describes locally advanced, technically unresectable tumor.

PART IV
Musculoskeletal Sites

21

Bone

(Primary malignant lymphoma and multiple myeloma are not included.)

C40.0	Long bones of upper limb, scapula, and associated joints	C40.8	Overlapping lesion of bones, joints, and articular cartilage of limbs	C41.4	Pelvic bones, sacrum, coccyx, and associated joints
C40.1	Short bones of upper limb and associated joints	C40.9	Bone of limb, NOS	C41.8	Overlapping lesion of bones, joints, and articular cartilage
C40.2	Long bones of lower limb and associated joints	C41.0	Bones of skull and face and associated joints	C41.9	Bone, NOS
C40.3	Short bones of lower limb and associated joints	C41.1	Mandible		
		C41.2	Vertebral column		
		C41.3	Rib, sternum, clavicle, and associated joints		

SUMMARY OF CHANGES

- T1 has changed from "Tumor confined within the cortex" to "Tumor 8 cm or less in greatest dimension."

- T2 has changed from "Tumor invades beyond the cortex" to "Tumor more than 8 cm in greatest dimension."

- T3 designation of skip metastasis is defined as "Discontinuous tumors in the primary bone site." This designation is a Stage III tumor that was not previously defined.

- M1 lesions have been divided into M1a and M1b.

- M1a is lung-only metastases.

- M1b is metastases to other distant sites, including lymph nodes.

- In the Stage Grouping, Stage IVA is M1a, and Stage IVB is M1b.

INTRODUCTION

This classification is used for all primary malignant tumors of bone except primary malignant lymphoma and multiple myeloma. Cases are categorized by histological type (e.g., osteosarcoma, chondrosacrcoma) and by histologic grade of differentiation.

ANATOMY

Primary Site. All bones of the skeleton.

Regional Lymph Nodes. Regional lymph node metastasis from bone tumors is extremely rare.

Metastatic Sites. A metastatic site includes any site beyond the regional lymph nodes of the primary site. Spread to the lungs is frequent.

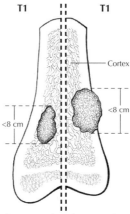

FIGURE 21.1. T1 is defined as tumor less than 8 cm in greatest dimension whether the tumor is confined within the cortex or invades beyond the cortex.

DEFINITIONS

Primary Tumor (T)

TX Primary tumor cannot be assessed
T0 No evidence of primary tumor
T1 Tumor 8 cm or less in greatest dimension (Figure 21.1)
T2 Tumor more than 8 cm in greatest dimension (Figure 21.2A, B)
T3 Discontinuous tumors in the primary bone site (Figure 21.3)

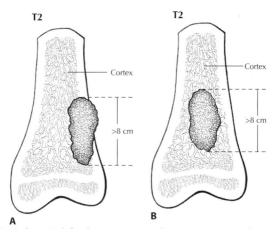

A   B

FIGURE 21.2. A. T2 is defined as tumor more than 8 cm in greatest dimension whether the tumor is confined within the cortex or invades beyond the cortex. **B.** T2 is defined as tumor more than 8 cm in greatest dimension whether the tumor is confined within the cortex or invades beyond the cortex.

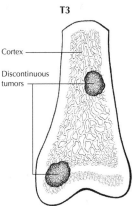

T3

Cortex

Discontinuous tumors

FIGURE 21.3. T3 is defined as discontinuous tumors in the primary bone site.

Regional Lymph Nodes (N)
NX   Regional lymph nodes cannot be assessed[1]
N0   No regional lymph node metastasis
N1   Regional lymph node metastasis

Distant Metastasis (M)
MX   Distant metastasis cannot be assessed
M0   No distant metastasis
M1   Distant metastasis
M1a   Lung (Figure 21.4)
M1b   Other distant sites (Figure 21.5)

Histologic Grade (G)
GX   Grade cannot be assessed
G1   Well differentiated—Low grade
G2   Moderately differentiated—Low grade
G3   Poorly differentiated—High grade
G4   Undifferentiated—High grade[2]

STAGE GROUPING

IA	T1	N0	M0	G1,2	Low grade
IB	T2	N0	M0	G1,2	Low grade
IIA	T1	N0	M0	G3,4	High grade
IIB	T2	N0	M0	G3,4	High grade
III	T3	N0	M0	Any G	
IVA	Any T	N0	M1a	Any G	
IVB	Any T	N1	Any M	Any G	
	Any T	Any N	M1b	Any G	

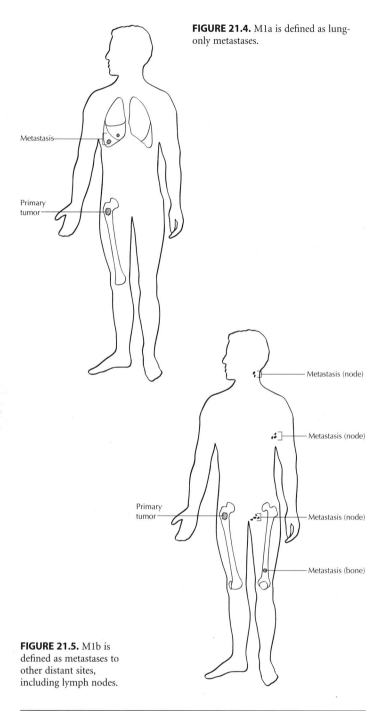

FIGURE 21.4. M1a is defined as lung-only metastases.

Metastasis

Primary tumor

Metastasis (node)

Metastasis (node)

Primary tumor

Metastasis (node)

Metastasis (bone)

FIGURE 21.5. M1b is defined as metastases to other distant sites, including lymph nodes.

1. Because of the rarity of lymph node involvement in sarcomas, the designation NX may not be appropriate and could be considered N0 if no clinical involvement is evident.
2. Ewing's sarcoma is classified as G4.

21

Soft Tissue Sarcoma

(Kaposi's sarcoma, dermatofibrosarcoma protuberans, fibromatosis [desmoid tumor], and sarcoma arising from the dura mater, brain, parenchymatous organs, or hollow viscera are not included.)

C38.0	Heart	C47.5	Peripheral nerves and autonomic nervous system of pelvis	C49.2	Connective, subcutaneous, and other soft tissues of lower limb and hip
C38.1	Anterior mediastinum				
C38.1	Posterior mediastinum	C47.6	Peripheral nerves and autonomic nervous system of trunk, NOS	C49.3	Connective, subcutaneous, and other soft tissues of thorax
C38.3	Mediastinum, NOS				
C38.8	Overlapping lesion of heart, mediastinum, and pleura	C47.8	Overlapping lesion of peripheral nerves and autonomic nervous system	C49.4	Connective, subcutaneous, and other soft tissues of abdomen
C47.0	Peripheral nerves and autonomic nervous system of head, face, and neck	C47.9	Autonomic nervous system, NOS	C49.5	Connective, subcutaneous, and other soft tissues of pelvis
		C48.0	Retroperitoneum		
C47.1	Peripheral nerves and autonomic nervous system of upper limb and shoulder	C48.1	Specified parts of peritoneum	C49.6	Connective, subcutaneous, and other soft tissues of trunk, NOS
		C48.2	Peritoneum, NOS		
		C48.8	Overlapping lesion of retroperitoneum and peritoneum	C49.7	Overlapping lesion of connective, subcutaneous, and other soft tissues
C47.2	Peripheral nerves and autonomic nervous system of lower limb and hip				
C47.3	Peripheral nerves and autonomic nervous system of thorax	C49.0	Connective, subcutaneous, and other soft tissues of head, face, and neck	C49.9	Connective, subcutaneous, and other soft tissues, NOS
C47.4	Peripheral nerves and autonomic nervous system of abdomen	C49.1	Connective, subcutaneous, and other soft tissues of upper limb and shoulder		

SUMMARY OF CHANGES

- Angiosarcoma and malignant mesenchymoma are no longer included in the list of histologic types for this site.

- Gastrointestinal stromal tumor and Ewing's sarcoma/primitive neuroectodermal tumor have been added to the list of histologic types for this site.

- Fibrosarcoma grade I has been replaced by fibromatosis (desmoid tumor) in the list of histologic types not included in this site.

- G 1–2, T2b, N0, M0 tumors have been reclassified as Stage I rather than Stage II disease.

22

INTRODUCTION

The staging system applies to all soft tissue sarcomas except Kaposi's sarcoma, dermatofibrosarcoma, infantile fibrosarcoma, and angiosarcoma. In addition, sarcomas arising within the confines of the dura mater, including the brain, and sarcomas arising in parenchymatous organs and from hollow viscera are not optimally staged by this system.

Data to support this staging system are based on current analyses from multiple institutions and represent the recommendations of an AJCC task force on soft tissue sarcoma. In the era of cytoreductive neoadjuvant treatments, clinical and pathologic staging may be altered in the future. Because pathologic staging drives adjuvant therapy decisions, patients should be restaged after neoadjuvant therapies have been administered.

Histologic type, grade, and tumor size and depth are essential for staging. Histologic grade of sarcoma is one of the most important parameters of the staging system. Grade is based on analysis of various pathologic features of a tumor, such as histologic subtype, degree of differentiation, mitotic activity, and necrosis. Accurate grading requires an adequate sample of well-fixed tissue for evaluation. Accurate grading is not always possible on the basis of needle biopsies or in tumors that have been previously irradiated or treated with chemotherapy.

The current staging system does not take into account anatomic site. However, anatomic site is known to influence outcome, and therefore outcome data should be reported specifying site. Generic grouping of site is accepted. The following site groups can be used in reports that include sarcomas arising in tissues other than soft tissues (such as parenchymal organs). Extremity and superficial trunk can be combined; viscera, including all the intra-abdominal viscera, can also be combined. Where enough numbers exist, these can be reported by subdivision into the various components of the gastrointestinal tract. Lung, gastrointestinal, genitourinary, and gynecologic sarcomas should be grouped separately.

Site Groups for Soft Tissue Sarcomas
Head and neck
Extremity and superficial trunk
Gastrointestinal
Genitourinary
Visceral
Retroperitoneal
Gynecologic
Breast
Lung, pleura, mediastinum
Other

STAGING OF SOFT TISSUE SARCOMA

Inclusions. The present staging system applies to soft tissue sarcomas. Primary sarcomas can arise from a variety of soft tissues. These tissues include fibrous connective tissue, fat, smooth or striated muscle, vascular tissue, peripheral neural tissue, and visceral tissue.

Regional Lymph Nodes. Involvement of regional lymph nodes by soft tissue sarcomas is uncommon in adults. When present, regional nodal disease has prognostic significance similar to that of visceral metastatic disease.

Metastatic Sites. Metastatic sites for soft tissue sarcoma are often dependent on the original site of the primary lesion. For example, the most common site

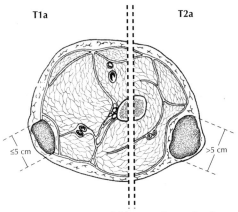

FIGURE 22.1. T1a is defined as a superficial tumor 5 cm or less in greatest dimension and T2a is defined as a superficial tumor more than 5 cm in greatest dimension.

of metastatic disease for patients with extremity sarcomas is the lung, whereas retroperitoneal and gastrointestinal sarcomas often have liver as the first site of metastasis.

DEFINITIONS

Primary Tumor (T)

TX   Primary tumor cannot be assessed
T0   No evidence of primary tumor
T1   Tumor 5 cm or less in greatest dimension
    T1a Superficial tumor[1] (Figure 22.1)
    T1b Deep tumor (Figure 22.2)
T2   Tumor more than 5 cm in greatest dimension
    T2a Superficial tumor[1] (Figure 22.1)
    T2b Deep tumor (Figure 22.3)

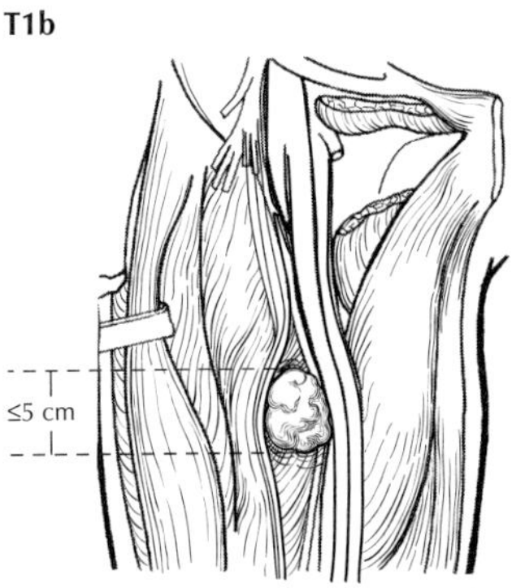

T1b

FIGURE 22.2. T1b is a deep tumor 5 cm or less in greatest dimension.

T2b

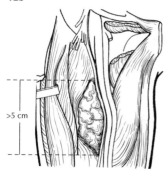

FIGURE 22.3. T2b is a deep tumor more than 5 cm in greatest dimension.

>5 cm

Regional Lymph Nodes (N)

NX   Regional lymph nodes cannot be assessed
N0   No regional lymph node metastasis
N1   Regional lymph node metastasis

Distant Metastasis (M)

MX   Distant metastasis cannot be assessed
M0   No distant metastasis
M1   Distant metastasis

Histologic Grade (G)

GX   Grade cannot be assessed
G1   Well differentiated
G2   Moderately differentiated
G3   Poorly differentiated
G4   Poorly differentiated or undifferentiated (four-tiered systems only)[2]

STAGE GROUPING

IA	T1a	N0	NX	M0	G1–2	G1	Low
	T1b	N0	NX	M0	G1–2	G1	Low
IB	T2a	N0	NX	M0	G1–2	G1	Low
	T2b	N0	NX	M0	G1–2	G1	Low
IIA	T1a	N0	NX	M0	G3–4	G2–3	High
	T1b	N0	NX	M0	G3–4	G2–3	High
IIB	T2a	N0	NX	M0	G3–4	G2–3	High
III	T2b	N0	NX	M0	G3–4	G2–3	High
IV	Any T	N1		M0	Any G	Any G	High or Low
	Any T	Any N		M1	Any G	Any G	High or Low

NOTES

1. Superficial tumor is located exclusively above the superficial fascia without invasion of the fascia; deep tumor is located either exclusively beneath the superficial fascia, superficial to the fascia with invasion of or through the fascia, or both superficial yet beneath the fascia. Retroperitoneal, mediastinal, and pelvic sarcomas are classified as deep tumors.
2. Ewing's sarcoma is classified as G4.

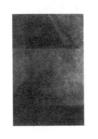

PART V
Skin

23

Carcinoma of the Skin
(Excluding Eyelid, Vulva, and Penis)

C44.0	Skin of lip, NOS	C44.5	Skin of trunk	C44.8	Overlapping lesion of
C44.2	External ear	C44.6	Skin of upper limb		skin
C44.3	Skin of other and		and shoulder	C44.9	Skin, NOS
	unspecified parts of	C44.7	Skin of lower limb	C63.2	Scrotum, NOS
	face		and hip		
C44.4	Skin of scalp and neck				

SUMMARY OF CHANGES

• The definitions of TNM and the Stage Groupings for this chapter have not changed from the Fifth Edition.

INTRODUCTION

This chapter applies to non-melanomatous cancers of the skin, which are predominantly basal cell carcinomas and squamous cell carcinomas. Skin cancers are largely related to solar exposure and are relatively common, although their frequency varies with geographical latitude and population at risk. For example, they occur in 729 individuals per 100,000 population in Hawaii but in only 195 per 100,000 in the northern United States. Higher rates are found in Australia and New Zealand, and the incidence generally is rising rapidly. Basal cell carcinomas are the most common cancer in humans, and are four to five times more common than squamous cell carcinomas of the skin. For the most part, non-melanomatous skin cancers have a good prognosis and nearly always can be treated with curative intent.

ANATOMY

Primary Site. The skin is made up of three layers: an outermost epidermis, a middle dermis, and an inner subcutis. The epidermis consists predominantly of stratified squamous epithelium, the outermost layer of which is keratinized. The innermost layer consists primarily of germinative cells and melanocytes. The dermis is made up of connective tissue and elastic fibers immersed in an amorphous matrix of mucoproteins and mucopolysaccharides. The subcutis is predominantly adipose tissue. The sebaceous and other glands of the skin, as well as the hair follicles—collectively called adnexal structures—are found in the dermis and subjacent subcutis. All of the components of the skin (epidermis, dermis, and adnexal structures within the subcutis) can give rise to malignant neoplasms.

Cancers of the skin most commonly arise on those surfaces exposed to sunlight (including the face, ears, hands, and scalp, especially in balding men) and the role of sunlight in the induction of cutaneous cancer has been well described. Approximately four-fifths of all cutaneous squamous cell cancers and approximately two-thirds of all basal cell cancers occur in unprotected sun-exposed skin of lightly pigmented persons. Squamous cell carcinoma can also arise in skin that was previously scarred or ulcerated—that is, at sites of burns and chronic ulcers. Radiation in other than ultraviolet forms, chemicals, and genetic syndromes are also proven causes of cutaneous carcinomas.

Skin cancers rarely cause symptoms. Signs vary depending on the local site of origin and whether the precursor lesion is an actinic keratosis or a cutaneous ulcer. Squamous cell tumors developing at the site of actinic keratoses usually begin as hyperkeratotic papules or plaques or as ulcers. Induration, which is usually absent in actinic keratoses, may develop early in squamous cell cancer. Further progression is associated with thickening of the plaque, ulceration, and bleeding. Tumors that arise in cutaneous ulcers or burn scars present as an expanding mass at the site. High-risk tumors (higher local recurrence rate or high risk for metastasis) are found on the lip, scalp, ears, eyelids, and nose.

Basal cell carcinomas initially appear clinically as firm, translucent papules coursed by telangiectatic blood vessels. Central areas of crusting and depression, associated with ulceration, usually occur late. Bleeding, however, may be described in early as well as late lesions. Pigmentation occurs uncommonly and may lead clinically to confusion with cutaneous melanoma. Morpheaform basal cell carcinoma (basal cell carcinoma with a fibrotic component) may look and feel like patches of scleroderma, or a scar, and is generally without telangiectasia or measurable elevation.

Primary Growth. Local extension is the predominant mode of growth of nonmelanomatous skin cancers. Basal cell carcinomas that remain untreated for long periods will eventually erode adjacent structures, such as bone, and into local vasculature. Perineural invasion in morpheaform basal cell cancers is often observed, and it is associated with a high rate of incomplete excision and recurrence. Squamous cell carcinoma may also penetrate into other local structures, including muscle, bone, and vasculature.

Regional Lymph Nodes. Skin cancers characteristically spread by local extension. Involvement of regional lymph nodes infrequently occurs and is usually associated with large size and invasiveness into the dermis and subcutaneous fat. Which specific lymph node chains are involved depends on the location of the primary lesion, because tumor cells are passively borne along with the "draining" lymphatic fluid, usually to the geographically closest node(s). Regional lymph node chains are illustrated in Figures 23.1, 23.2, and 23.3. In this context,

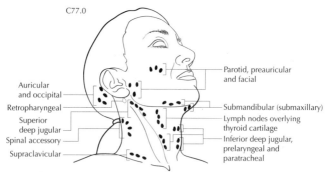

FIGURE 23.1. C77.0, regional lymph nodes of the head and neck.

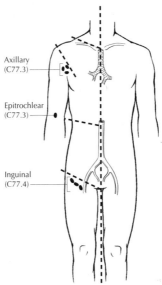

FIGURE 23.2. C77.3, axillary and epitrochlear lymph nodes, and C77.4, inguinal lymph nodes.

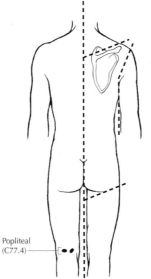

FIGURE 23.3. C77.4, popliteal lymph nodes.

Tis

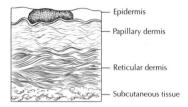

FIGURE 23.4. Carcinoma *in situ*.

— Epidermis

— Papillary dermis

— Reticular dermis

— Subcutaneous tissue

for tumors of the lower torso or lower extremities, the inguinal nodes are considered the regional basin and should be designated N1. For pN (pathologic staging), histologic examination of a regional lymphadenectomy specimen should include careful examination of all resected nodes.

Hematogenously Borne Metastases. Basal cell and squamous cell cancers that arise in actinically damaged skin are relatively slow growing and rarely metastasize. Metastases are more likely to arise from squamous cell tumors that originate in scars or ulcers. Tumors that metastasize have often been present for a long time before metastases are observed. The most common visceral metastatic site is the lung, especially for squamous cell carcinomas. Other sites of distant spread are unusual. Non-melanoma skin cancers arising in transplant patients may be more aggressive and may metastasize more readily and more widely.

DEFINITIONS

Primary Tumor (T)

TX   Primary tumor cannot be assessed
T0   No evidence of primary tumor
Tis   Carcinoma *in situ* (Figure 23.4)
T1   Tumor 2 cm or less in greatest dimension (Figure 23.5)
T2   Tumor more than 2 cm, but not more than 5 cm, in greatest dimension (Figure 23.6)

T1

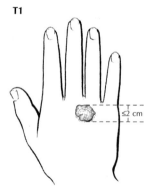

≤2 cm

FIGURE 23.5. T1 is defined as a tumor 2 cm or less in greatest dimension.

FIGURE 23.6. T2 is defined as a tumor more than 2 cm, but not more than 5 cm, in greatest dimension.

T2

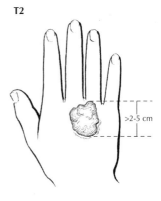

>2-5 cm

T3   Tumor more than 5 cm in greatest dimension (Figure 23.7)

T4   Tumor invades deep extradermal structures (i.e., cartilage, skeletal muscle, or bone) (Figure 23.8)

Note: In case of multiple simultaneous tumors, the tumor with the highest T category will be classified and the number of separate tumors will be indicated in parentheses, e.g., T2 (5) (Figure 23.9).

T3

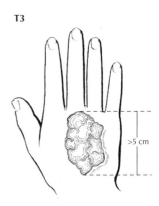

>5 cm

FIGURE 23.7. T3 is defined as a tumor more than 5 cm in greatest dimension.

23

T4

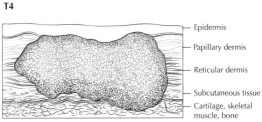

Epidermis

Papillary dermis

Reticular dermis

Subcutaneous tissue

Cartilage, skeletal muscle, bone

FIGURE 23.8. T4 is defined as tumor invading deep extradermal structures such as cartilage, skeletal muscle, or bone.

T2(5)

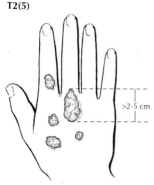

>2-5 cm

FIGURE 23.9. In the case of multiple simultaneous tumors, the tumor with the highest T category will be classified and the number of separate tumors indicated in parentheses.

Regional Lymph Nodes (N)

NX Regional lymph nodes cannot be assessed
N0 No regional lymph node metastasis
N1 Regional lymph node metastasis

Distant Metastasis (M)

MX Distant metastasis cannot be assessed
M0 No distant metastasis
M1 Distant metastasis

Figure 23.10 illustrates the designation of N1 (Stage III disease) based upon metastasis to regional lymph nodes vs. the designation of M1 (Stage IV disease) defined by distant metastasis, in this case to lymph nodes outside the region of the primary tumor. Figures 23.11, 23.12, 23.13, and 23.14 illustrate N1 (Stage

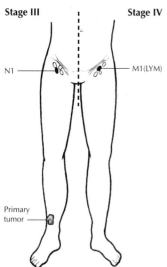

Stage III   Stage IV

N1 ——   —— M1(LYM)

Primary tumor ——

FIGURE 23.10. N1 disease is defined as regional lymph node metastasis while M1 disease involves distant metastasis (here to lymph nodes beyond the region of the primary tumor).

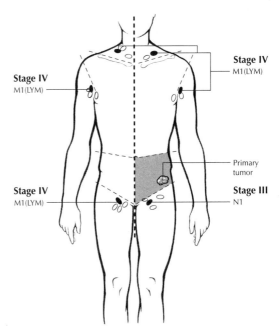

FIGURE 23.11. Stage of disease as determined by lymph node involvement relative to the location of the primary tumor. The shaded areas indicate involvement of regional lymph nodes or N1 disease (Stage III). Nonshaded areas indicate distant metastasis to lymph nodes outside the primary tumor or M1 disease (Stage IV).

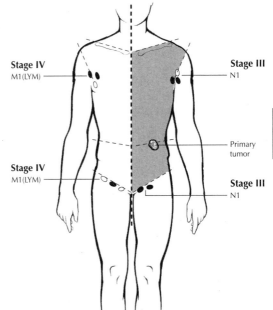

FIGURE 23.12. Stage of disease as determined by lymph node involvement relative to the location of the primary tumor. The shaded areas indicate involvement of regional lymph nodes or N1 disease (Stage III). Nonshaded areas indicate distant metastasis to lymph nodes outside the primary tumor or M1 disease (Stage IV).

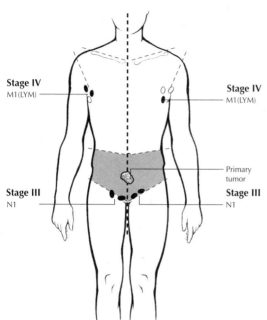

FIGURE 23.13.
Stage of disease as determined by lymph node involvement relative to the location of the primary tumor. The shaded areas indicate involvement of regional lymph nodes or N1 disease (Stage III). Nonshaded areas indicate distant metastasis to lymph nodes outside the primary tumor or M1 disease (Stage IV).

Stage IV
M1(LYM)

Stage IV
M1(LYM)

Primary tumor

Stage III
N1

Stage III
N1

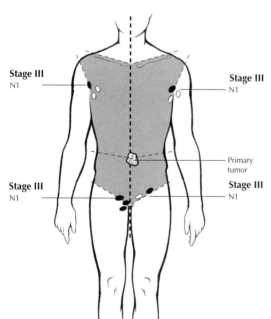

FIGURE 23.14.
Stage of disease as determined by lymph node involvement relative to the location of the primary tumor. The shaded areas indicate involvement of regional lymph nodes or N1 disease (Stage III). Metastasis to either the axillary or inguinal lymph nodes are both considered N1 (Stage III) disease due to the location of the primary tumor directly in the center of the torso.

Stage III
N1

Stage III
N1

Primary tumor

Stage III
N1

Stage III
N1

III) or M1 (Stage IV) disease based upon whether affected lymph nodes fall within or beyond the regional nodal chain of the primary tumor. The shaded areas in the figures indicate disease spread to regional lymph nodes for a classification of N1 (Stage III).

STAGE GROUPING

0	Tis	N0	M0
I	T1	N0	M0
II	T2	N0	M0
	T3	N0	M0
III	T4	N0	M0
	Any T	N1	M0
IV	Any T	Any N	M1

Melanoma of the Skin

C44.0	Skin of lip, NOS	C44.7	Skin of lower limb	C51.9	Vulva, NOS
C44.1	Eyelid		and hip	C60	Penis
C44.2	External ear	C44.8	Overlapping lesion of	C60.0	Prepuce
C44.3	Skin of other and		skin	C60.1	Glans penis
	unspecified parts of	C44.9	Skin, NOS	C60.2	Body of penis
	face	C51	Vulva	C60.8	Overlapping lesion of
C44.4	Skin of scalp and	C51.0	Labium majus		penis
	neck	C51.1	Labium minus	C60.9	Penis, NOS
C44.5	Skin of trunk	C51.2	Clitoris	C63.2	Scrotum, NOS
C44.6	Skin of upper limb	C51.8	Overlapping lesion of		
	and shoulder		vulva		

SUMMARY OF CHANGES

- Melanoma thickness and ulceration, but not level of invasion, are used in the T category (except for T1 melanomas).

- The number of metastatic lymph nodes, rather than their gross dimensions, and the delineation of clinically occult (i.e., microscopic) vs. clinically apparent (i.e., macroscopic) nodal metastases are used in the N category.

- The site of distant metastases and the presence of elevated serum lactic dehydrogenase (LDH) are used in the M category.

- All patients with Stage I, II, or III disease are upstaged when a primary melanoma is ulcerated.

- Satellite metastases around a primary lesion and in-transit metastases have been merged into a single staging entity that is grouped Stage IIIc disease.

- A new convention for defining clinical and pathologic staging has been developed that takes into account the new staging information gained from intra-operative lymphatic mapping and sentinel node excision.

INTRODUCTION

Melanoma of the skin continues to increase in frequency, with 47,700 new cases and 9,200 deaths expected in 2005 (1). Melanoma can arise from skin anywhere on the body. It occurs most commonly in fair-skinned persons, especially those with a history of significant sun exposure.

A completely revised melanoma staging system is provided herein, along with operational definitions. In addition, a major database analysis of prognostic factors involving 17,600 cancer patients from 13 cancer centers and organizations was performed to validate the staging categories and groupings (2). Within each stage grouping and its subgroups, there is a uniform risk for distant metastases and a uniform survival probability. This revised version of melanoma staging more accurately reflects the prognosis and natural history of melanoma and will therefore be more applicable to treatment planning and clinical trials involving melanoma.

ANATOMY

Primary Sites. Cutaneous melanoma can occur anywhere on the skin. It occurs most commonly on the extremities in females and on the trunk in males. Melanomas located on the palms, soles, and nailbeds (acral lentiginous melanoma), although they occur infrequently, are distinctive because they can occur in individuals of any ethnic origin and in persons with no history of significant sun exposure.

Regional Lymph Nodes. The regional lymph nodes are the most common site of metastases. The widespread use of cutaneous lymphoscintigraphy, lymphatic mapping, and sentinel lymph node biopsies has greatly enhanced the ability to identify the presence or absence of, and to stage, nodal metastases. Intralymphatic regional metastases may also become clinically manifest either as satellite metastases (defined arbitrarily as intralymphatic metastases occurring within 2 cm of the primary melanoma) or as in-transit metastases (defined arbitrarily as intralymphatic metastases occurring more than 2 cm from the primary melanoma but before the first echelon of regional lymph nodes). By convention, the term regional nodal metastases refers to disease confined to one nodal basin or two contiguous nodal basins, as in patients with nodal disease in combinations of femoral/iliac, axillary/supraclavicular, cervical/supraclavicular, axillary/femoral, or bilateral axillary or femoral metastases.

Metastatic Sites. Melanoma can metastasize to virtually any organ site. Metastases most commonly occur in the skin or soft tissues, the lung, and the liver.

DEFINITIONS

Primary Tumor (T)

TX   Primary tumor cannot be assessed (e.g., shave biopsy or regressed melanoma)
T0   No evidence of primary tumor
Tis   Melanoma *in situ*
T1   Melanoma ≤1.0 mm with or without ulceration (Figures 24.1A–D)
T1a   Melanoma ≤1.0 mm in thickness and level II or III, no ulceration (Figure 24.2)
T1b   Melanoma ≤1.0 mm in thickness and level IV or V or with ulceration (Figures 24.3A, B)
T2   Melanoma 1.01–2.0 mm in thickness with or without ulceration
T2a   Melanoma 1.01–2.0 mm in thickness, no ulceration (Figure 24.4)
T2b   Melanoma 1.01–2.0 mm in thickness, with ulceration (Figure 24.5)
T3   Melanoma 2.01–4.0 mm in thickness with or without ulceration
T3a   Melanoma 2.01–4.0 mm in thickness, no ulceration (Figure 24.6)
T3b   Melanoma 2.01–4.0 mm in thickness, with ulceration (Figure 24.7)
T4   Melanoma greater than 4.0 mm in thickness with or without ulceration
T4a   Melanoma >4.0 mm in thickness, no ulceration (Figure 24.8)
T4b   Melanoma >4.0 mm in thickness, with ulceration (Figure 24.9)

Regional Lymph Nodes (N)

NX   Regional lymph nodes cannot be assessed
N0   No regional lymph node metastasis

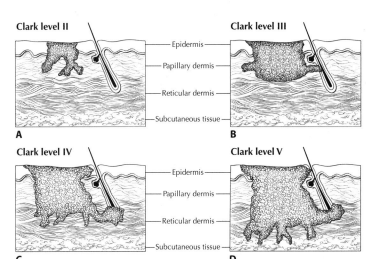

FIGURE 24.1. A–D. The level of invasion, as defined by Dr. Wallace Clark, is used to define subcategories of T1 melanomas but not for thicker melanomas (i.e., T2, T3, or T4). **A–D** illustrate Clark levels II, III, IV, and V, respectively.

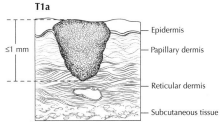

FIGURE 24.2. T1a is defined as melanoma ≤1.0 mm in thickness, level II or III, with no ulceration.

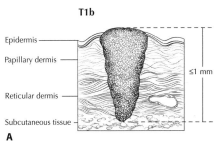

FIGURE 24.3. A. T1b is defined as melanoma ≤1.0 mm in thickness, level IV or V, or with ulceration. This figure illustrates T1b with level V invasion and no ulceration.

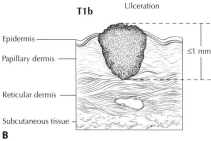

FIGURE 24.3. B. T1b is illustrated here as melanoma ≤1.0 mm in thickness with level II invasion and ulceration.

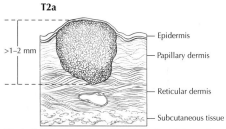

FIGURE 24.4. T2a is defined as melanoma greater than 1.0 mm but not more than 2.0 mm in thickness without ulceration.

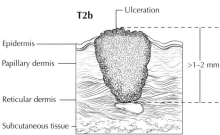

FIGURE 24.5. T2b is defined as melanoma greater than 1.0 mm but not more than 2.0 mm in thickness with ulceration.

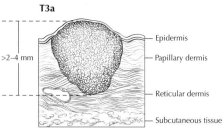

FIGURE 24.6. T3a is defined as melanoma greater than 2.0 mm but not more than 4.0 mm in thickness without ulceration.

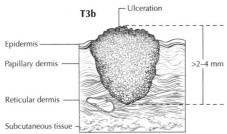

FIGURE 24.7. T3b is defined as melanoma greater than 2.0 mm but not more than 4.0 mm in thickness with ulceration.

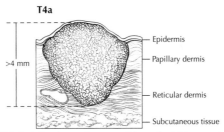

FIGURE 24.8. T4a is defined as melanoma >4.0 mm in thickness without ulceration.

N1   Metastasis in one lymph node

N1a   Clinically occult (microscopic) metastasis (Figure 24.10)

N1b   Clinically apparent (macroscopic) metastasis (Figure 24.11)

N2   Metastasis in 2 to 3 regional nodes or intralymphatic regional metastasis without nodal metastasis

N2a   Clinically occult (microscopic) metastasis (Figure 24.12)

N2b   Clinically apparent (macroscopic) metastasis (Figure 24.13)

N2c   Satellite or in-transit metastasis without nodal metastasis (Figure 24.14)

N3   Metastasis in four or more regional nodes, or matted metastatic nodes, or in-transit metastasis or satellite(s) with metastasis in regional node(s) (Figure 24.15)

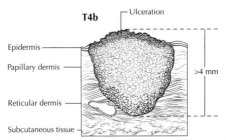

FIGURE 24.9. T4b is defined as melanoma >4.0 mm in thickness with ulceration.

N1a

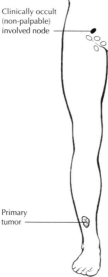

Clinically occult
(non-palpable)
involved node

Primary
tumor

FIGURE 24.10. N1a is defined as clinically occult metastasis in one lymph node.

N1b

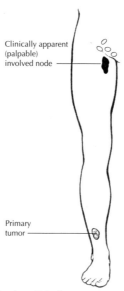

Clinically apparent
(palpable)
involved node

Primary
tumor

FIGURE 24.11. N1b is defined as clinically apparent metastasis in one lymph node.

N2a

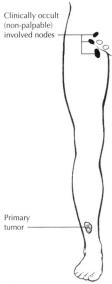

Clinically occult
(non-palpable)
involved nodes

Primary
tumor

FIGURE 24.12. N2a is defined as clinically occult metastasis in 2–3 regional nodes.

N2b

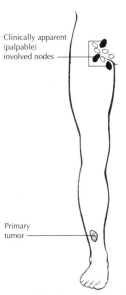

Clinically apparent
(palpable)
involved nodes

Primary
tumor

24

FIGURE 24.13. N2b is defined as clinically apparent metastasis in 2–3 regional lymph nodes.

N2c

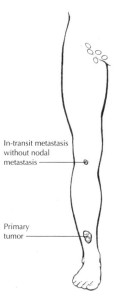

In-transit metastasis without nodal metastasis

Primary tumor

FIGURE 24.14. N2c is defined as satellite or in-transit metastasis without nodal metastasis. This figure illustrates an in-transit metastasis, which is defined as intralymphatic metastasis occurring more than 2 cm from the primary melanoma but before the first echelon of regional lymph nodes.

N3

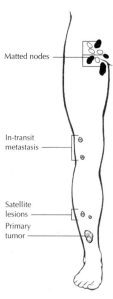

Matted nodes

In-transit metastasis

Satellite lesions

Primary tumor

FIGURE 24.15. N3 may be defined as metastasis in 4 or more regional nodes or matted metastatic nodes (top) or as in-transit metastasis (middle) or satellite lesions that occur within 2 cm of the primary tumor (bottom).

Distant Metastasis (M)

MX Distant metastasis cannot be assessed

M0 No distant metastasis

M1 Distant metastasis

M1a Metastasis to skin, subcutaneous tissues, or distant lymph nodes

M1b Metastasis to lung

M1c Metastasis to all other visceral sites or distant metastasis at any site associated with an elevated serum lactic dehydrogenase (LDH)

PATHOLOGIC STAGE GROUPING[1]

0	Tis	N0	M0
IA	T1a	N0	M0
IB	T1b	N0	M0
	T2a	N0	M0
IIA	T2b	N0	M0
	T3a	N0	M0
IIB	T3b	N0	M0
	T4a	N0	M0
IIC	T4b	N0	M0
IIIA	T1-4a	N1a	M0
	T1-4a	N2a	M0
IIIB	T1-4b	N1a	M0
	T1-4b	N2a	M0
	T1-4a	N1b	M0
	T1-4a	N2b	M0
	T1-4a/b	N2c	M0
IIIC	T1-4b	N1b	M0
	T1-4b	N2b	M0
	Any T	N3	M0
IV	Any T	Any N	M1

CLINICAL STAGE GROUPING[2]

0	Tis	N0	M0
IA	T1a	N0	M0
IB	T1b	N0	M0
	T2a	N0	M0
IIA	T2b	N0	M0
	T3a	N0	M0
IIB	T3b	N0	M0
	T4a	N0	M0
IIC	T4b	N0	M0
III	Any T	N1	M0
	Any T	N2	M0
	Any T	N3	M0
IV	Any T	Any N	M1

24

NOTES

1. Pathologic staging includes microstaging of the primary melanoma and pathologic information about the regional lymph nodes after partial or complete lymphadenectomy. Pathologic Stage 0 or Stage IA patients are the exception; they do not require pathological evaluation of their lymph nodes.
2. Clinical staging includes microstaging of the primary melanoma and clinical/radiologic evaluation for metastases. By convention, it should be used after complete excision.

REFERENCES

1. Jemal A, Taylor M, Ward E, et al. Cancer statistics, 2005. CA Cancer J Clin 55:10–30, 2005.
2. Balch C, Soong SJ, Gershenwald JE, Thompson JF, Reintgen DS, Cascinelli N, Urist MM, McMasters KM, Ross MI, Kirkwood JM, Atkins MB, Thompson JA, Coit DG, Byrd D, Desmond R, Zhang Y, Liu PY, Lyman GH, Morabito A. Prognostic factors analysis of 17,600 melanoma patients: Validation of the AJCC melanoma staging system. J Clin Oncol 19:3622–3634, 2001.

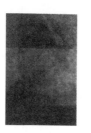

PART VI
Breast

25

Breast

C50.0	Nipple	C50.4	Upper outer quadrant of breast	C50.8	Overlapping lesion of breast
C50.1	Central portion of the breast	C50.5	Lower outer quadrant of breast	C50.9	Breast, NOS
C50.2	Upper inner quadrant of breast	C50.6	Axillary tail of breast		
C50.3	Lower inner quadrant of breast				

SUMMARY OF CHANGES

- Micrometastases are distinguished from isolated tumor cells on the basis of size and histologic evidence of malignant activity.

- Identifiers have been added to indicate the use of sentinel lymph node dissection and immunohistochemical or molecular techniques.

- Major classifications of lymph node status are designated according to the number of involved axillary lymph nodes as determined by routine hematoxylin and eosin staining (preferred method) or by immunohistochemical staining.

- The classification of metastasis to the infraclavicular lymph nodes has been added as N3.

- Metastasis to the internal mammary nodes, based on the method of detection and the presence or absence of axillary nodal involvement, has been reclassified. Microscopic involvement of the internal mammary nodes detected by sentinel node dissection using lymphoscintigraphy but not by imaging studies or clinical examination is classified as N1. Macroscopic involvement of the internal mammary nodes as detected by imaging studies (excluding lymphoscintigraphy) or by clinical examination is classified as N2 if it occurs in the absence of metastases to the axillary lymph nodes or as N3 if it occurs in the presence of metastases to the axillary lymph nodes.

- Metastasis to the supraclavicular lymph nodes has been reclassified as N3 rather than M1.

INTRODUCTION

This staging system for carcinoma of the breast applies to infiltrating (including microinvasive) and *in situ* carcinomas. Microscopic confirmation of the diagnosis is mandatory, and the histologic type and grade of carcinomas should be recorded

ANATOMY

Primary Site. The anatomic subsites of the breast are illustrated in Figure 25.1. The mammary gland, situated on the anterior chest wall, is composed of glandular tissue with a dense fibrous stroma. The glandular tissue consists of lobules that group together into 15–25 lobes arranged approximately in a spoke-like pattern. Multiple major and minor ducts connect the milk-secreting lobular units to the nipple. Small milk ducts course throughout the breast, converging into larger collecting ducts that open into the lactiferous sinus at the base of the nipple. Most cancers form initially in the terminal duct lobular units of the breast. Glandular tissue is more abundant in the upper outer portion of the breast; as a result, half of all breast cancers occur in this area.

Chest Wall. The chest wall includes ribs, intercostal muscles and serratus anterior muscle, but not the pectoral muscles.

Regional Lymph Nodes. The regional lymph nodes of the breast are illustrated in Figure 25.2. The breast lymphatics drain by way of three major routes: axillary, transpectoral, and internal mammary. Intramammary lymph nodes are coded as axillary lymph nodes for staging purposes. Supraclavicular lymph nodes are classified as regional lymph nodes for staging purposes. Metastasis to any other lymph node, including cervical or contralateral internal mammary lymph nodes, is classified as distant (M1).

The regional lymph nodes are as follows:

1. Axillary (ipsilateral): interpectoral (Rotter's) nodes and lymph nodes along the axillary vein and its tributaries that may be (but are not required to be) divided into the following levels:
   a. Level I (low-axilla): lymph nodes lateral to the lateral border of pectoralis minor muscle.
   b. Level II (mid-axilla): lymph nodes between the medial and lateral borders of the pectoralis minor muscle and the interpectoral (Rotter's) lymph nodes.
   c. Level III (apical axilla): lymph nodes medial to the medial margin of the pectoralis minor muscle, including those designated as apical.
2. Internal mammary (ipsilateral): lymph nodes in the intercostal spaces along the edge of the sternum in the endothoracic fascia.
3. Supraclavicular: lymph nodes in the supraclavicular fossa, a triangle defined by the omohyoid muscle and tendon (lateral and superior border), the

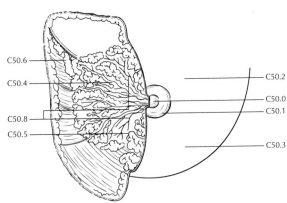

FIGURE 25.1. Anatomic sites and subsites of the breast.

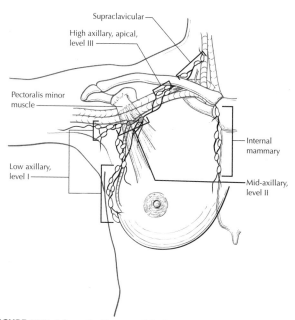

FIGURE 25.2. Schematic diagram of the breast and regional lymph nodes.

internal jugular vein (medial border), and the clavicle and subclavian vein (lower border). Adjacent lymph nodes outside of this triangle are considered to be lower cervical nodes (M1).

Metastatic Sites. Tumor cells may be disseminated by either the lymphatic or the blood vascular system. The four major sites of involvement are bone, lung, brain, and liver, but tumor cells are also capable of metastasizing to many other sites.

DEFINITIONS

Primary Tumor (T)

Definitions for classifying the primary tumor (T) are the same for clinical and for pathologic classification. If the measurement is made by physical examination, the examiner will use the major headings (T1, T2, or T3). If other measurements, such as mammographic or pathologic measurements, are used, the subsets of T1 can be used. Tumors should be measured to the nearest 0.1 cm increment.

TX	Primary tumor cannot be assessed
T0	No evidence of primary tumor
Tis	Carcinoma *in situ*
Tis	(DCIS) Ductal carcinoma *in situ*
Tis	(LCIS) Lobular carcinoma *in situ*
Tis	(Paget's) Paget's disease of the nipple with no tumor (Figure 25.3)

25

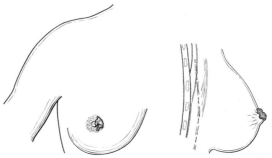

FIGURE 25.3. Tis (Paget's) is defined as Paget's disease of the nipple with no tumor.

Note: Paget's disease associated with a tumor is classified according to the size of the tumor.

T1	Tumor 2 cm or less in greatest dimension
T1mic	Microinvasion 0.1 cm or less in greatest dimension (Figure 25.4)
T1a	Tumor more than 0.1 cm but not more than 0.5 cm in greatest dimension (Figure 25.5)
T1b	Tumor more than 0.5 cm but not more than 1 cm in greatest dimension (Figure 25.5)
T1c	Tumor more than 1 cm but not more than 2 cm in greatest dimension (Figure 25.5)
T2	Tumor more than 2 cm but not more than 5 cm in greatest dimension (Figure 25.6)

T1mic(m) or T1mic(3)

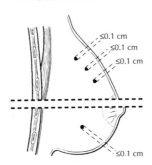

T1mic

FIGURE 25.4. T1mic is defined as microinvasion 0.1 cm or less in greatest dimension. The presence of multiple tumor foci of microinvasion (top of diagram) should be noted in parentheses.

T1

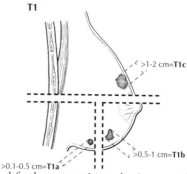

>1-2 cm=**T1c**

>0.5-1 cm=**T1b**

>0.1-0.5 cm=**T1a**

FIGURE 25.5. T1 is defined as a tumor 2 cm or less in greatest dimension. T1a is defined as tumor more than 0.1 cm but not more than 0.5 cm in greatest dimension; T1b is defined as tumor more than 0.5 cm but not more than 1 cm in greatest dimension; T1c is defined as tumor more than 1 cm but not more than 2 cm in greatest dimension.

T3	Tumor more than 5 cm in greatest dimension (Figure 25.6)
T4	Tumor of any size with direct extension to
	a. Chest wall or
	b. Skin, only as described below
T4a	Extension to chest wall, not including pectoralis muscle (Figure 25.7)
T4b	Edema (including peau d'orange) or ulceration of the skin of the breast, or satellite skin nodules confined to the same breast (Figures 25.8A, B)
T4c	Both T4a and T4b (Figure 25.9)
T4d	Inflammatory carcinoma (Figure 25.10)

T2

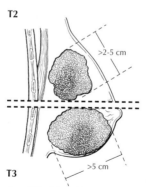

>2-5 cm

>5 cm

T3

FIGURE 25.6. T2 (above dotted line) is defined as tumor more than 2 cm but not more than 5 cm in greatest dimension and T3 (below dotted line) is defined as tumor more than 5 cm in greatest dimension.

25

T4a

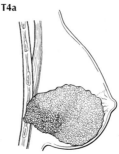

FIGURE 25.7. T4 is defined as a tumor of any size with direct extension to chest wall, not including pectoralis muscle.

T4b   **T4b**

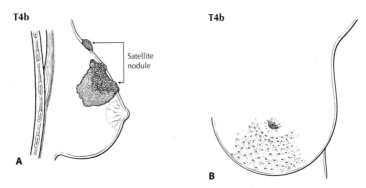

Satellite
nodule

A

B

FIGURE 25.8. A. T4b, illustrated here as satellite skin nodules, is defined as edema (including peau d'orange) or ulceration of the skin of the breast, or satellite skin nodules confined to the same breast. **B.** T4b illustrated here as edema (including peau d'orange).

T4c

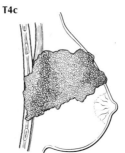

FIGURE 25.9. T4c is defined as both T4a and T4b.

T4d

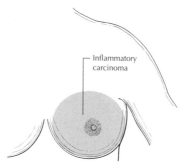

FIGURE 25.10. T4d, inflammatory carcinoma.

Regional Lymph Nodes (N)

NX   Regional lymph nodes cannot be assessed (e.g., previously removed)

N0   No regional lymph node metastasis

N1   Metastasis in movable ipsilateral axillary lymph node(s) (Figure 25.11)

N2   Metastases in ipsilateral axillary lymph nodes fixed or matted, or in clinically apparent[1] ipsilateral internal mammary nodes in the *absence* of clinically evident axillary lymph node metastasis

N2a   Metastasis in ipsilateral axillary lymph nodes fixed to one another (matted) or to other structures (Figure 25.12)

N2b   Metastasis only in clinically apparent[1] ipsilateral internal mammary nodes and in the *absence* of clinically evident axillary lymph node metastasis (Figure 25.13)

N3   Metastasis in ipsilateral infraclavicular lymph node(s) with or without axillary lymph node involvement, or in clinically apparent[1] ipsilateral

N1

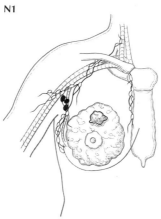

FIGURE 25.11. N1 is defined as metastasis in movable ipsilateral axillary lymph node(s).

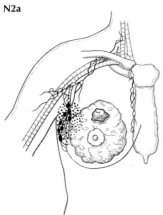

N2a

FIGURE 25.12. N2a is defined as metastasis in ipsilateral axillary lymph nodes fixed to one another (matted) or to other structures.

internal mammary lymph node(s) and in the *presence* of clinically evident axillary lymph node metastasis; or metastasis in ipsilateral supraclavicular lymph node(s) with or without axillary or internal mammary lymph node involvement

N3a Metastasis in ipsilateral infraclavicular lymph node(s) (Figure 25.14)
N3b Metastasis in ipsilateral internal mammary lymph node(s) and axillary lymph node(s) (Figure 25.15)
N3c Metastasis in ipsilateral supraclavicular lymph node(s) (Figure 25.16)

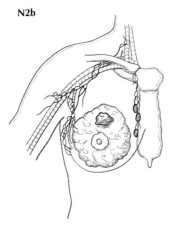

N2b

FIGURE 25.13. N2b is defined as metastasis only in clinically apparent[1] ipsilateral internal mammary nodes and in the *absence* of clinically evident axillary lymph node metastasis.

FIGURE 25.14. N3a metastasis in ipsilateral infraclavicular lymph node(s) without axillary or internal mammary lymph node involvement.

N3a

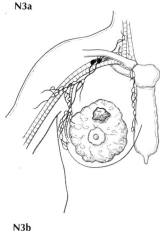

N3b

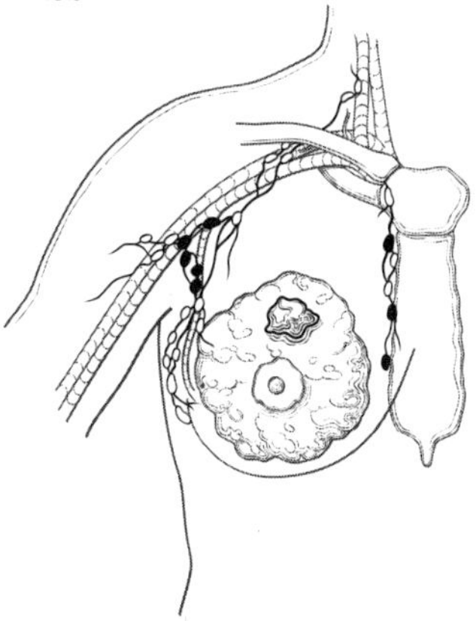

FIGURE 25.15. N3b metastasis in ipsilateral internal mammary lymph node(s) and axillary lymph node(s).

pN3c

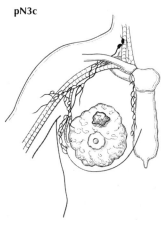

FIGURE 25.16. N3c is defined as metastasis in ipsilateral supraclavicular lymph node(s).

25

Regional Lymph Nodes (pN)[2]

pNX   Regional lymph nodes cannot be assessed (e.g., previously removed, or not removed for pathologic study)

pN0   No regional lymph node metastasis histologically, no additional examination for isolated tumor cells (ITC)[3]

pN0(i−)   No regional lymph node metastasis histologically, negative IHC

pN0(i+)   No regional lymph node metastasis histologically, positive IHC, no IHC cluster greater than 0.2 mm (Figure 25.17)

pN0(mol−)   No regional lymph node metastasis histologically, negative molecular findings (RT-PCR)[4]

pN0(mol+)   No regional lymph node metastasis histologically, positive molecular findings (RT-PCR)[4]

pN1   Metastasis in 1 to 3 axillary lymph nodes, and/or in internal mammary nodes with microscopic disease detected by sentinel lymph node dissection but not clinically apparent[5]

pN1mi   Micrometastasis (greater than 0.2 mm, none greater than 2.0 mm) (Figure 25.18)

pN1a   Metastasis in 1 to 3 axillary lymph nodes (Figure 25.18)

pN1b   Metastasis in internal mammary nodes with microscopic disease detected by sentinel lymph node dissection but not clinically apparent[5] (Figure 25.19)

pN1c   Metastasis in 1 to 3 axillary lymph nodes and in internal mammary lymph nodes with microscopic disease detected by sentinel lymph node dissection but not clinically apparent[5,6] (Figure 25.20)

pN2   Metastasis in 4 to 9 axillary lymph nodes, or in clinically apparent[1] internal mammary lymph nodes in the *absence* of axillary lymph node metastasis

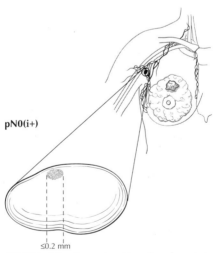

pN0(i+)

≤0.2 mm

FIGURE 25.17. pN0(i+) is defined as regional lymph node metastasis histologically, positive IHC, no IHC cluster greater than 0.2 mm.

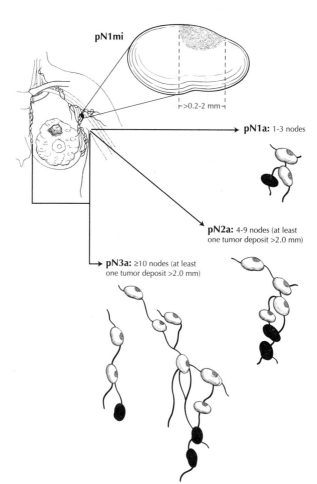

FIGURE 25.18. Illustrated definition of pN1mi, defined as micrometastasis greater than 0.2 mm with none greater than 2.0 mm, as well as pN1a, pN2a, and pN3a.

pN2a	Metastasis in 4 to 9 axillary lymph nodes (at least one tumor deposit greater than 2.0 mm) (Figure 25.18)
pN2b	Metastasis in clinically apparent[1] internal mammary lymph nodes in the *absence* of axillary lymph node metastasis (Figure 25.21)
pN3	Metastasis in 10 or more axillary lymph nodes, or in infraclavicular lymph nodes, or in clinically apparent[1] ipsilateral internal mammary lymph nodes in the *presence* of 1 or more positive axillary lymph nodes; or in more than 3 axillary lymph nodes with clinically negative microscopic metastasis in internal mammary lymph nodes; or in ipsilateral supraclavicular lymph nodes

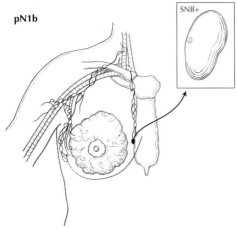

FIGURE 25.19. pN1b with isolated tumor cells in a single internal mammary node, sentinel lymph node positive.

pN3a   Metastasis in 10 or more axillary lymph nodes (at least one tumor deposit greater than 2.0 mm), or metastasis to the infraclavicular lymph nodes (Figure 25.18)

pN3b   Metastasis in clinically apparent[1] ipsilateral internal mammary lymph nodes in the *presence* of 1 or more positive axillary lymph nodes; or in more than 3 axillary lymph nodes and in internal mammary lymph nodes with microscopic disease detected by

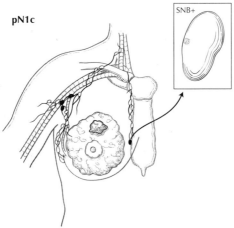

FIGURE 25.20. pN1c illustrating 3 positive axillary lymph nodes with isolated tumor cells in a single internal mammary lymph node, sentinel lymph node positive.

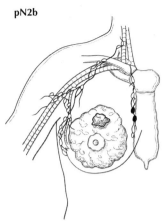

pN2b

FIGURE 25.21. pN2b illustrating clinically apparent metastasis in 2 positive internal mammary nodes with no axillary lymph node involvement.

> sentinel lymph node dissection but not clinically apparent[5] (Figure 25.22A, B)

pN3c   Metastasis in ipsilateral supraclavicular lymph nodes (Figure 25.16)

Distant Metastasis (M)

MX   Distant metastasis cannot be assessed
M0   No distant metastasis
M1   Distant metastasis

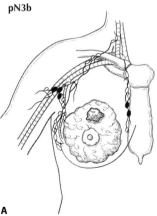

pN3b

A

FIGURE 25.22. A. pN3b illustrated as clinically apparent metastasis in 2 positive internal mammary nodes in the presence of 3 positive axillary lymph nodes.

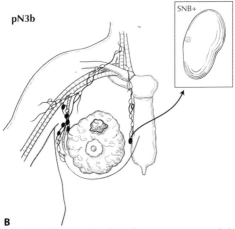

pN3b

SNB+

FIGURE 25.22. B. pN3b illustrated as clinically apparent metastasis in 6 positive axillary lymph nodes with isolated tumor cells in one internal mammary lymph node, sentinel lymph node positive.

STAGE GROUPING

0	Tis	N0	M0
I	T1[7]	N0	M0
IIA	T0	N1	M0
	T1[7]	N1	M0
	T2	N0	M0
IIB	T2	N1	M0
	T3	N0	M0
IIIA	T0	N2	M0
	T1[7]	N2	M0
	T2	N2	M0
	T3	N1	M0
	T3	N2	M0
IIIB	T4	N0	M0
	T4	N1	M0
	T4	N2	M0
IIIC	Any T	N3	M0
IV	Any T	Any N	M1

Note: Stage designation may be changed if post-surgical imaging studies reveal the presence of distant metastases, provided that the studies are carried out within 4 months of diagnosis in the absence of disease progression and provided that the patient has not received neoadjuvant therapy.

NOTES

1. *Clinically apparent* is defined as detected by imaging studies (excluding lymphoscintigraphy) or by clinical examination or grossly visible pathologically.

2. Classification is based on axillary lymph node dissection with or without sentinel lymph node dissection. Classification based solely on sentinel lymph node dissection without subsequent axillary lymph node dissection is designated (sn) for "sentinel node," e.g., pNO(i+)(sn).

3. Isolated tumor cells (ITC) are defined as single tumor cells or small cell clusters not greater than 0.2 mm, usually detected only by immunohistochemical (IHC) or molecular methods but which may be verified on H&E stains. ITCs do not usually show evidence of metastatic activity (e.g., proliferation or stromal reaction).

4. RT-PCR: reverse transcriptase/polymerase chain reaction.

5. *Not clinically apparent* is defined as not detected by imaging studies (excluding lymphoscintigraphy) or by clinical examination.

6. If associated with greater than 3 positive axillary lymph nodes, the internal mammary nodes are classified as pN3b to reflect increased tumor burden.

7. T1 includes T1mic.

25

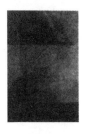

PART VII
Gynecologic Sites

26

Vulva

(Mucosal malignant melanoma is not included.)

C51.0	Labium majus	C51.8	Overlapping lesion of
C51.1	Labium minus		vulva
C51.2	Clitoris	C51.9	Vulva, NOS

SUMMARY OF CHANGES

• The definitions of TNM and the Stage Grouping for this chapter have not changed from the Fifth Edition.

ANATOMY

Primary Site. The vulva is the anatomic site immediately external to the vagina. It includes the labia and the perineum. The tumor may extend to involve the vagina, urethra, or anus. It may be fixed to the pubic bone (Figure 26.1).

Regional Lymph Nodes. (See Chapter 27, Figure 27.3.) The femoral and inguinal nodes are the sites of regional spread. For pN, histologic examination of an inguinal lymphadenectomy specimen will ordinarily include six or more lymph nodes. Negative pathologic examination of a lesser number of nodes still mandates a pN0 designation. The concept of sentinel lymph node mapping where only one or two key nodes are removed is currently being investigated.

Metastatic Sites. The metastatic sites include any site beyond the area of the regional lymph nodes. Tumor involvement of pelvic lymph nodes, including internal iliac, external iliac, and common iliac lymph nodes, is considered distant metastasis.

DEFINITIONS

The definitions of the T categories correspond to the stages accepted by the Federation Internationale de Gynecologie et d'Obstetrique (FIGO). Both systems are included for comparison.

Primary Tumor (T)

TNM	FIGO	Definitions
Categories	Stages	
TX		Primary tumor cannot be assessed
T0		No evidence of primary tumor
Tis	0	Carcinoma *in situ* (preinvasive carcinoma)
T1	I	Tumor confined to the vulva or vulva and perineum, 2 cm or less in greatest dimension (Figure 26.2)

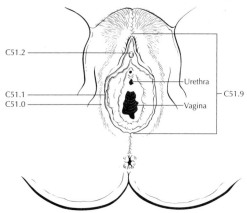

FIGURE 26.1. Anatomic sites and subsites of the vulva.

T1a	IA	Tumor confined to the vulva or vulva and perineum, 2 cm or less in greatest dimension, and with stromal invasion no greater than 1 mm[1] (Figure 26.3A)
T1b	IB	Tumor confined to the vulva or vulva and perineum, 2 cm or less in greatest dimension, and with stromal invasion greater than 1 mm[1] (Figure 26.3B)
T2	II	Tumor confined to the vulva or vulva and perineum, more than 2 cm in greatest dimension (Figure 26.4)
T3	III	Tumor of any size with contiguous spread to the lower urethra and/or vagina or anus (Figures 26.5A, B)

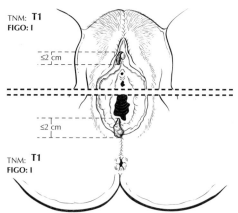

FIGURE 26.2. T1 tumor confined to the vulva (top of figure, above dotted line) or vulva and perineum (bottom of figure, below dotted line), 2 cm or less in greatest dimension.

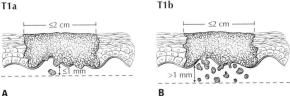

T1a   **T1b**

A   **B**

FIGURE 26.3. T1a **A** is tumor confined to the vulva or vulva and perineum, 2 cm or less in greatest dimension, and with stromal invasion no greater than 1 mm.[1] T1b **B** is tumor confined to the vulva or vulva and perineum, 2 cm or less in greatest dimension, and with stromal invasion greater than 1 mm.[1]

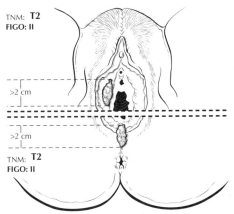

FIGURE 26.4. T2 tumor confined to the vulva (top of figure, above dotted line) or vulva and perineum (bottom of figure, below dotted line) more than 2 cm in greatest dimension.

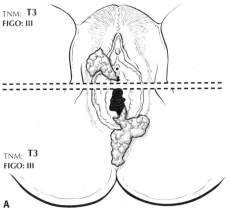

A

FIGURE 26.5. A. T3 is a tumor of any size with contiguous spread to the lower urethra (top of figure, above dotted line) or vagina and/or anus (bottom of figure, below dotted line).

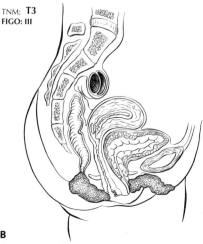

TNM: **T3**
FIGO: III

B

FIGURE 26.5. B. Cross-sectional diagram showing spread of tumor into anus and lower urethra.

T4   IVA   Tumor invades any of the following: upper urethra, bladder mucosa, rectal mucosa, or is fixed to the pubic bone (Figure 26.6)

Regional Lymph Nodes (N)
NX   Regional lymph nodes cannot be assessed
N0   No regional lymph node metastasis

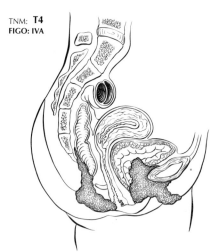

TNM: **T4**
FIGO: IVA

FIGURE 26.6. T4 is defined as tumor invading any of the following: upper urethra, bladder mucosa, rectal mucosa, or is fixed to the pubic bone.

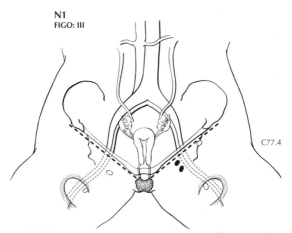

FIGURE 26.7. N1: unilateral regional lymph node metastasis.

| N1 | III | Unilateral regional lymph node metastasis (Figure 26.7) |
| N2 | IVA | Bilateral regional lymph node metastasis (Figure 26.8) |

Every effort should be made to determine the site and laterality of lymph node metastases. However, if "regional lymph node metastases, NOS" is the final diagnosis, then the patient should be staged as N1.

Distant Metastasis (M)

MX		Distant metastasis cannot be assessed
M0		No distant metastasis
M1	IVB	Distant metastasis (including pelvic lymph node metastasis)

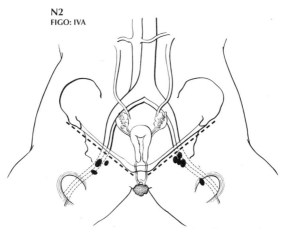

FIGURE 26.8. N2: bilateral regional lymph node metastasis.

STAGE GROUPING (AJCC/UICC/FIGO)

0	Tis	N0	M0
I	T1	N0	M0
IA	T1a	N0	M0
IB	T1b	N0	M0
II	T2	N0	M0
III	T1	N1	M0
	T2	N1	M0
	T3	N0	M0
	T3	N1	M0
IVA	T1	N2	M0
	T2	N2	M0
	T3	N2	M0
	T4	Any N	M0
IVB	Any T	Any N	M1

NOTE

1. The depth of invasion is defined as the measurement of the tumor from the epithelial-stromal junction of the adjacent most superficial dermal papilla to the deepest point of invasion.

Vagina

C52.9   Vagina, NOS

SUMMARY OF CHANGES

- The definitions of TNM and the Stage Grouping for this chapter have not changed from the Fifth Edition.

ANATOMY

Primary Site. The vagina extends from the vulva upward to the uterine cervix. It is lined by squamous epithelium with only rare glandular structures. The vagina (Figure 27.1) is drained by lymphatics toward the pelvic nodes (Figure 27.2) in its upper two-thirds and toward the inguinal nodes (Figure 27.3) in its lower third.

Regional Lymph Nodes. The upper two-thirds of the vagina is drained by lymphatics to the pelvic nodes, including:

Obturator
Internal iliac (hypogastric)
External iliac
Pelvic, NOS

The lower third of the vagina is drained to the groin nodes, including:

Inguinal
Femoral

Metastatic Sites. The most common sites of distant spread include the aortic lymph nodes, lungs, and skeleton.

DEFINITIONS

The definitions of the T categories correspond to the stages accepted by the Federation Internationale de Gynecologie et d'Obstetrique (FIGO). Both systems are included for comparison.

Primary Tumor (T)

TNM	FIGO	Definitions
Categories	Stages	
TX		Primary tumor cannot be assessed
T0		No evidence of primary tumor
Tis	0	Carcinoma *in situ*
T1	I	Tumor confined to vagina (Figure 27.4)
T2	II	Tumor invades paravaginal tissues but not to pelvic wall (Figure 27.5)

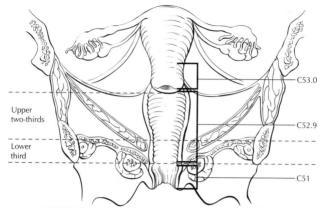

FIGURE 27.1. Anatomical sites and subsites of the vagina.

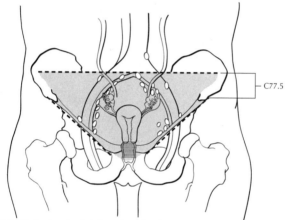

FIGURE 27.2. Regional pelvic lymph nodes draining the upper two-thirds of the vagina.

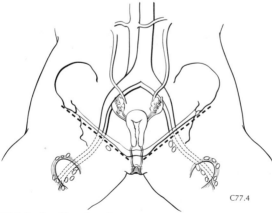

FIGURE 27.3. Regional lymph nodes in the groin draining the lower third of the vagina.

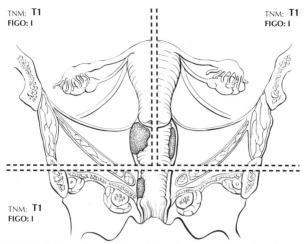

FIGURE 27.4. Three views of T1, each showing tumor confined to the vagina.

| T3 | III | Tumor extends to pelvic wall[1] (Figure 27.6) |
| T4 | IVA | Tumor invades mucosa of the bladder or rectum and/or extends beyond the true pelvis (bullous edema is not sufficient evidence to classify a tumor as T4) (Figure 27.7) |

Regional Lymph Nodes (N)

NX Regional lymph nodes cannot be assessed

N0 No regional lymph node metastasis

N1 Pelvic or inguinal lymph node metastasis (Figures 27.8A–C)

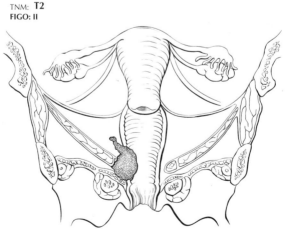

FIGURE 27.5. T2 tumor invading paravaginal tissues but not to pelvic wall.

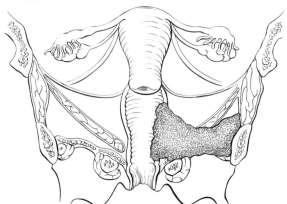

FIGURE 27.6. T3 tumor extending to pelvic wall.

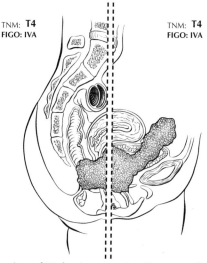

FIGURE 27.7. Two views of T4 showing tumor invading rectum (left side of dotted line) or extending beyond true pelvis or invading bladder (right side of dotted line).

FIGURE 27.8. A–C. N1: pelvic (27.8A) or unilateral inguinal (27.8B) or bilateral inguinal (27.8C) lymph node metastasis.

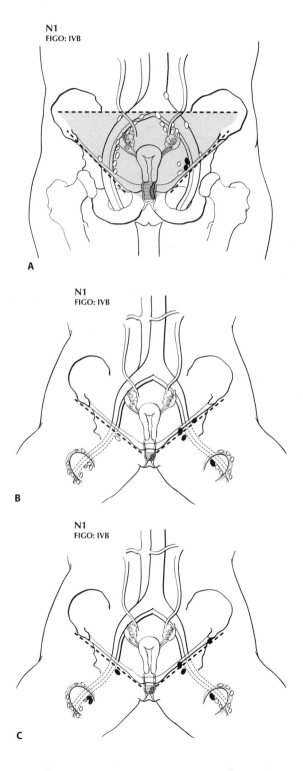

A

B

C

Distant Metastasis (M)

MX   Distant metastasis cannot be assessed
M0   No distant metastasis
M1   IVB   Distant metastasis

STAGE GROUPING (AJCC/UICC/FIGO)

0	Tis	N0	M0
I	T1	N0	M0
II	T2	N0	M0
III	T1–T3	N1	M0
	T3	N0	M0
IVA	T4	Any N	M0
IVB	Any T	Any N	M1

NOTE

1. Pelvic wall is defined as the muscle, fascia, associated neurovascular structures, or skeletal portions of the bony pelvis.

Cervix Uteri

C53.0	Endocervix	C53.8	Overlapping lesion of	C53.9	Cervix uteri
C53.1	Exocervix		cervix uteri		

SUMMARY OF CHANGES
- The definitions of TNM and the Stage Grouping for this chapter have not changed from the Fifth Edition.

ANATOMY

Primary Site. The cervix is in the lower third of the uterus. It is roughly cylindrical in shape and projects into the upper vagina. Through the cervix runs the endocervical canal, which is the passageway connecting the vagina with the uterine cavity. The endocervical canal is lined by glandular or columnar epithelium. The vaginal portion of the cervix, known as the exocervix, is covered by squamous epithelium. The squamocolumnar junction is usually located at the external cervical os, where the endocervical canal begins. Cancer of the cervix may originate from the squamous epithelium of the exocervix or the glandular epithelium of the canal (Figure 28.1).

Regional Lymph Nodes. The cervix is drained by parametrial, cardinal, and uterosacral ligament routes into the following regional lymph nodes (Figure 28.2):

Parametrial
Paracervical
Obturator
Internal iliac (hypogastric)
External iliac
Common iliac
Sacral
Presacral

Metastatic Sites. The most common sites of distant spread include the aortic and mediastinal nodes, lungs, and skeleton. Para-aortic node involvement is considered distant metastasis and is coded M1.

DEFINITIONS

The definitions of the T categories correspond to the stages accepted by the Federation Internationale de Gynecologie et d'Obstetrique (FIGO). Both systems are included for comparison.

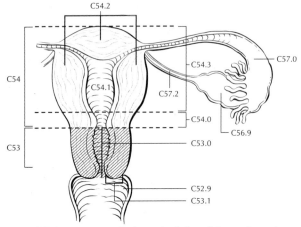

FIGURE 28.1. Anatomic sites and subsites of the cervix uteri.

Primary Tumor (T)

TNM Categories	FIGO Stages	Definitions
TX		Primary tumor cannot be assessed
T0		No evidence of primary tumor
Tis	0	Carcinoma *in situ*

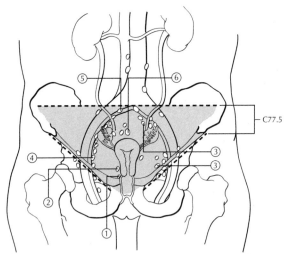

FIGURE 28.2. Regional lymph nodes of the cervix: (1) paracervical; (2) parametrial; (3) hypogastric (internal iliac) including obturator; (4) external iliac; (5) common iliac; (6) presacral.

T1	I	Cervical carcinoma confined to uterus (extension to corpus should be disregarded)
T1a	IA	Invasive carcinoma diagnosed only by microscopy.[1] All macroscopically visible lesions—even with superficial invasion— are T1b/IB. Stromal invasion with a maximal depth of 5.0 mm measured from the base of the epithelium and a horizontal spread of 7.0 mm or less. Vascular space involvement, venous or lymphatic, does not affect classification. (Figure 28.3)
T1a1	IA1	Measured stromal invasion 3.0 mm or less in depth and 7.0 mm or less in horizontal spread (Figure 28.4)
T1a2	IA2	Measured stromal invasion more than 3.0 mm and not more than 5.0 mm with a horizontal spread 7.0 mm or less (Figure 28.5)
T1b	IB	Clinically visible lesion confined to the cervix or microscopic lesion greater than T1a2/IA2 (Figure 28.6)
T1b1	IB1	Clinically visible lesion 4.0 cm or less in greatest dimension (Figure 28.7)
T1b2	IB2	Clinically visible lesion more than 4.0 cm in greatest dimension (Figure 28.8)
T2	II	Cervical carcinoma invades beyond uterus but not to pelvic wall or to lower third of vagina (Figure 28.9)
T2a	IIA	Tumor without parametrial invasion (Figure 28.9)
T2b	IIB	Tumor with parametrial invasion (Figure 28.9)
T3	III	Tumor extends to pelvic wall and/or involves lower third of vagina and/or causes hydronephrosis or nonfunctioning kidney (Figure 28.10)
T3a	IIIA	Tumor involves lower third of vagina, no extension to pelvic wall (Figure 28.10)

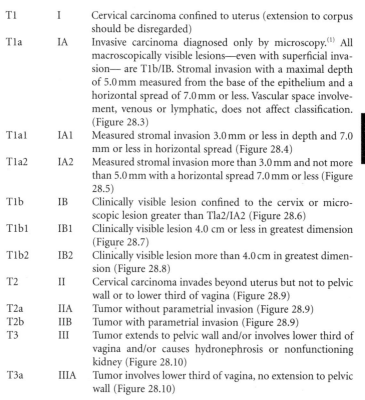

TNM: **T1a**
FIGO: IA

Invasive carcinoma diagnosed only by microscopy

FIGURE 28.3. T1a is defined as invasive carcinoma diagnosed only by microscopy[1] with stromal invasion to a maximal depth of 5.0 mm measured from the base of the epithelium and a horizontal spread of 7.0 mm or less.

TNM: **T1a1**
FIGO: IA1

Invasive carcinoma diagnosed only by microscopy

FIGURE 28.4. T1a1 is defined as invasive carcinoma diagnosed only by microscopy with measured stromal invasion 3.0 mm or less in depth and 7.0 mm or less in horizontal spread **B**.

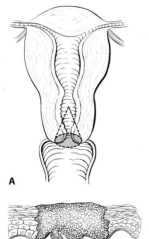

A

≤3 mm

B ←— ≤7 mm —→

TNM: **T1a2**
FIGO: IA2

Invasive carcinoma diagnosed only by microscopy

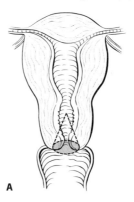

A

FIGURE 28.5. T1a2 is defined as invasive carcinoma diagnosed only by microscopy with measured stromal invasion more than 3.0 mm and not more than 5.0 mm with horizontal spread 7.0 mm or less **B**.

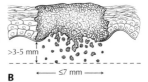

>3-5 mm

B ←— ≤7 mm —→

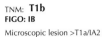

TNM: **T1b**
FIGO: IB

Microscopic lesion >T1a/IA2

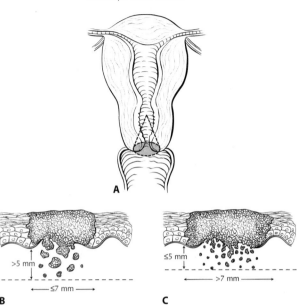

FIGURE 28.6. T1b is defined as a microscopic lesion greater than T1a2/IA2, i.e., stromal invasion greater than 5.0 mm and/or horizontal spread greater than 7.0 mm **B** and **C** or a clinically visible lesion confined to the cervix.

TNM: **T1b1**
FIGO: IB1

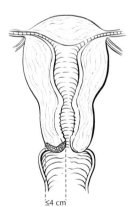

FIGURE 28.7. T1b1 is defined as a clinically visible lesion 4.0 cm or less in greatest dimension.

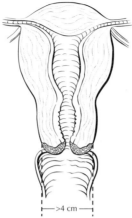

TNM: **T1b2**
FIGO: IB2

├─ >4 cm ─┤

FIGURE 28.8. T1b2 is defined as a clinically visible lesion more than 4.0 cm in greatest dimension.

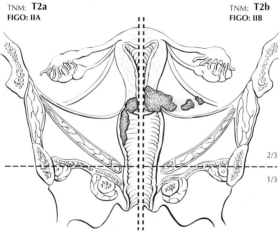

TNM: **T2a**
FIGO: IIA

TNM: **T2b**
FIGO: IIB

2/3

1/3

FIGURE 28.9. T2 is defined as a cervical carcinoma that invades beyond uterus but not to pelvic wall or to lower third of vagina. T2a (left of the vertical dotted line) is T2 tumor without parametrial invasion. T2b (right of the vertical dotted line) is T2 tumor with parametrial invasion.

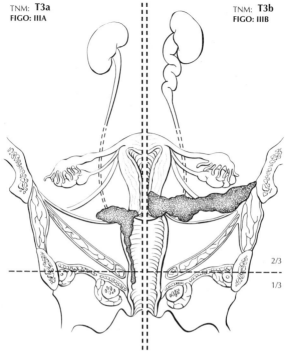

FIGURE 28.10. T3 tumor extends to pelvic wall and/or involves lower third of vagina and/or causes hydronephrosis or nonfunctioning kidney. T3a (left of vertical dotted line) involves lower third of vagina with no extension to pelvic wall. T3b (right of vertical dotted line) extends to pelvic wall and/or causes hydronephrosis or nonfunctioning kidney.

T3b	IIIB	Tumor extends to pelvic wall and/or causes hydronephrosis or nonfunctioning kidney (Figure 28.10)
T4	IVA	Tumor invades mucosa of bladder or rectum and/or extends beyond true pelvis (bullous edema is not sufficient evidence to classify a tumor as T4) (Figure 28.11)

Regional Lymph Nodes (N)

NX	Regional lymph nodes cannot be assessed
N0	No regional lymph node metastasis
N1	Regional lymph mode metastasis (Figure 28.12)

Distant Metastasis (M)

MX		Distant metastasis cannot be assessed
M0		No distant metastasis
M1	IVB	Distant metastasis

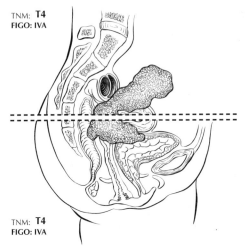

FIGURE 28.11. Two views of T4. Bottom of illustration (below dotted line), tumor invades mucosa of bladder or rectum. Top of illustration (above dotted line), tumor extends beyond true pelvis.

N1

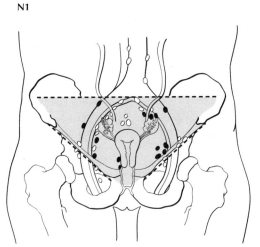

FIGURE 28.12. N1 is defined as regional lymph node metastasis.

STAGE GROUPING (AJCC/UICC/FIGO)

0	Tis	N0	M0
I	T1	N0	M0
IA	T1a	N0	M0
IA1	T1a1	N0	M0
IA2	T1a2	N0	M0
IB	T1b	N0	M0
IB1	T1b1	N0	M0
IB2	T1b2	N0	M0
II	T2	N0	M0
IIA	T2a	N0	M0
IIB	T2b	N0	M0
III	T3	N0	M0
IIIA	T3a	N0	M0
IIIB	T1	N1	M0
	T2	N1	M0
	T3a	N1	M0
	T3b	Any N	M0
IVA	T4	Any N	M0
IVB	Any T	Any N	M1

NOTE

1. The depth of invasion is defined as the measurement of the tumor from the epithelial-stromal junction of the adjacent most superficial dermal papilla to the deepest point of invasion.

Corpus Uteri

C54.0	Isthmus uteri	C45.3	Fundus uteri	C54.9	Corpus uteri
C54.1	Endometrium	C54.8	Overlapping lesion of	C55.9	Uterus, NOS
C54.2	Myometrium		corpus uteri		

SUMMARY OF CHANGES

· The definitions of TNM and the Stage Grouping for this chapter have not changed from the Fifth Edition.

ANATOMY

Primary Site. The upper two-thirds of the uterus above the level of the internal cervical os is referred to as the uterine corpus (see Figure 28.1). The oviducts (fallopian tubes) and the round ligaments enter the uterus at the upper and outer corners (cornu) of the pear-shaped organ. The portion of the uterus that is above a line connecting the tubo-uterine orifices is referred to as the uterine fundus. The lower third of the uterus is called the cervix and lower uterine segment. Tumor involvement of the endocervical mucosa and/or the stroma of the endocervix is prognostically important and affects staging (T2). The location of the tumor must be carefully evaluated and recorded by the pathologist. The depth of tumor invasion into the myometrium is also of prognostic significance and should be included in the pathology report. Extension of the tumor through the myometrial wall of the uterus into the parametrium occurs on occasion and constitutes regional extension (T3a). Involvement of the ovaries (T3a) by direct extension or metastases or extension to the vagina (T3b) occurs relatively infrequently.

Regional Lymph Nodes. The regional lymph nodes are paired and each of the paired sites should be examined. The regional nodes are illustrated in Figure 28.2 (see labels 2, 3, 4, 5, and 6) plus the para-aortic lymph nodes and regional lymph nodes, NOS.

Obturator
Internal iliac (hypogastric)
External iliac
Common iliac
Para-aortic
Presacral
Parametrial
Pelvic lymph nodes, NOS

For adequate evaluation of the regional lymph nodes, sampling of para-aortic and bilateral obturator nodes and at least one other regional node group should be documented in either or both of the operative and surgical pathology reports.

Parametrial nodes are not commonly detected unless a radical hysterectomy is performed for cases with gross cervical stromal invasion.

Metastatic Sites. The vagina and lung are the common metastatic sites. Intra-abdominal metastases occur frequently in advanced disease.

DEFINITIONS

Primary Tumor (T)

The definitions of the T categories correspond to the stages accepted by FIGO. FIGO stages are further subdivided by histologic grade of tumor—for example, Stage IC G2. Both systems are included for comparison.

FIGO recommends surgical/pathologic staging. Clinical staging is done with 1971 FIGO as follows:

TNM	FIGO	Definitions
cTis	0	Carcinoma *in situ*; histologic findings suspicious of malignancy
cT1	I	Carcinoma is confined to the corpus including the isthmus
cT1a	IA	Length of the uterine cavity is 8 cm or less
cT1b	IB	Length of the uterine cavity is more than 8 cm

Stage I cases should be subgrouped with regard to the histologic type of the adeno-carcinoma as follows:

G1		Highly differentiated adenomatous carcinoma
G2		Moderately differentiated adenomatous carcinoma with partly solid areas
G3		Predominately solid or entirely undifferentiated carcinoma
cT2	II	Carcinoma has involved the corpus and the cervix, but has not extended outside the uterus
cT3	III	Carcinoma has extended outside the uterus, but not outside the true pelvis
cT4	IV	Carcinoma has extended outside the true pelvis or has obviously involved the mucosa of the bladder or rectum (bullous edema as such does not permit a case to be allotted to stage IV)
cT4a	IVA	Spread of the growth to adjacent organs as urinary bladder, rectum, sigmoid colon, or small bowel

Stage 0 cases should not be included in any therapeutic statistics.

Primary Tumor (T)

TNM	FIGO	Definitions
TX		Primary tumor cannot be assessed
T0		No evidence of primary tumor
Tis	0	Carcinoma *in situ*
T1	I	Tumor confined to corpus uteri
T1a	IA	Tumor limited to endometrium (Figure 29.1)
T1b	IB	Tumor invades less than one-half of the myometrium (Figure 29.1)

Figure 29.1. T1 tumor confined to corpus uteri. T1a tumor is limited to endometrium (left); T1b tumor invades less than one-half of the myometrium (upper right); T1c tumor invades one-half or more of the myometrium (lower right) indicated by the tumor traversing the dotted horizontal line marking the halfway plane of the myometrium.

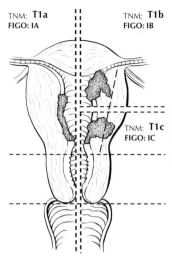

T1c	IC	Tumor invades one-half or more of the myometrium (Figure 29.1)
T2	II	Tumor invades cervix but does not extend beyond uterus (Figure 29.2)
T2a	IIA	Tumor limited to the glandular epithelium of the endocervix, with no evidence of connective tissue stromal invasion (Figure 29.2)
T2b	IIB	Invasion of the stromal connective tissue of the cervix (Figure 29.2)

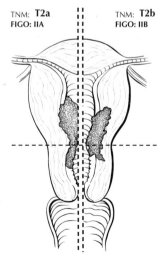

Figure 29.2. T2 tumor invades cervix but does not extend beyond uterus. T2a (left) is T2 tumor limited to the glandular epithelium of the endocervix with no evidence of connective tissue stromal invasion. T2b (right) is T2 tumor that has invaded the stromal connective tissue of the cervix.

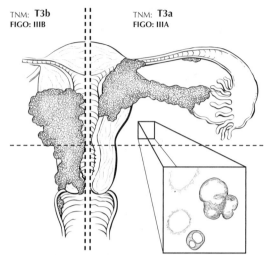

Figure 29.3. T3a (right) is a tumor involving serosa and/or adnexa (by direct extension or metastasis) and/or cancer cells in ascites or peritoneal washings. T3b (left) is a tumor with vaginal involvement (by direct extension or metastasis).

T3	III	Local and/or regional spread as defined below
T3a	IIIA	Tumor involves serosa and/or adnexa (direct extension or metastasis) and/or cancer cells in ascites or peritoneal washings (Figure 29.3)
T3b	IIIB	Vaginal involvement (direct extension or metastasis) (Figure 29.3)
T4	IVA	Tumor invades bladder mucosa and/or bowel mucosa (bullous edema is not sufficient evidence to classify a tumor as T4) (Figure 29.4)

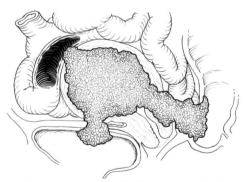

Figure 29.4. T4 tumor that invades bladder mucosa and/or bowel mucosa.

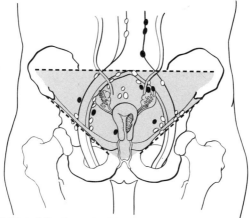

29

Figure 29.5. N1 is defined as regional lymph node metastasis to pelvic and/or para-aortic lymph nodes.

Regional Lymph Nodes (N)

NX		Regional lymph nodes cannot be assessed
N0		No regional lymph node metastasis
N1	IIIC	Regional lymph node metastasis to pelvic and/or para-aortic lymph nodes (Figure 29.5)

Distant Metastasis (M)

MX		Distant metastasis cannot be assessed
M0		No distant metastasis
M1	IVB	Distant metastasis includes metastasis to intra-abdominal lymph nodes other than para-aortic, and/or inguinal lymph nodes; excludes metastasis to vagina, pelvic serosa, or adnexa

STAGE GROUPING(AJCC/UICC/FIGO)

0	Tis	N0	M0
I	T1	N0	M0
IA	T1a	N0	M0
IB	T1b	N0	M0
IC	T1c	N0	M0
II	T2	N0	M0
IIA	T2a	N0	M0
IIB	T2b	N0	M0
III	T3	N0	M0
IIIA	T3a	N	M0
IIIB	T3b	N0	M0

IIIC	T1	N1	M0
	T2	N1	M0
	T3	N1	M0
IVA	T4	Any N	M0
IVB	Any T	Any N	M1

30

Ovary

C56.9   Ovary

SUMMARY OF CHANGES

• The definitions of TNM and the Stage Grouping for this chapter have not changed from the Fifth Edition.

ANATOMY

30

Primary Site. The ovaries are a pair of solid, flattened ovoids, 2 to 4 cm in diameter that are connected by a peritoneal fold to the broad ligament and by the infundibulopelvic ligament to the lateral wall of the pelvis. They are attached medially to the uterus by the utero-ovarian ligament. (See Figure 28.1.)

In some cases, an adenocarcinoma is primary in the peritoneum. The ovaries are not involved or are only involved with minimal surface implants. The clinical presentation, surgical therapy, chemotherapy, and prognosis of these peritoneal tumors mirror those of papillary serous carcinoma of the ovary. Patients who undergo prophylactic oophorectomy for a familial history of ovarian cancer appear to retain a 1 to 2% chance of developing peritoneal adenocarcinoma, which is histopathologically and clinically similar to primary ovarian cancer.

Regional Lymph Nodes. The lymphatic drainage occurs by the utero-ovarian and round ligament trunks and an external iliac accessory route into the following regional nodes:

External iliac
Internal iliac (hypogastric)
Obturator
Sacral
Common iliac
Para-aortic
Inguinal
Pelvic, NOS
Retroperitoneal, NOS

For pN0, histologic examination should include both pelvic and para-aortic lymph nodes. Figure 30.1 illustrates the regional lymph nodes.

Metastatic Sites. The peritoneum, including the omentum and the pelvic and abdominal visceral and parietal peritoneum, comprises common sites for seeding. Diaphragmatic and liver surface involvement are also common. However, to be consistent with FIGO staging, these implants within the abdominal cavity (T3) are not considered distant metastases. Primary peritoneal adenocarcinoma is always metastatic at diagnosis (M1). Extraperitoneal sites,

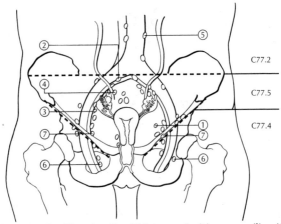

FIGURE 30.1. Regional lymph nodes: (1) hypogastric; (2) common iliac; (3) external iliac; (4) lateral sacral; (5) para-aortic; (6) inguinal; (7) obturator.

including parenchymal liver, lung, skeletal metastases, and supraclavicular and axillary nodes, are M1.

DEFINITIONS

Primary Tumor (T)

TNM Categories	FIGO Stages	Definitions
TX		Primary tumor cannot be assessed
T0		No evidence of primary tumor
T1	I	Tumor limited to ovaries (one or both)
T1a	IA	Tumor limited to one ovary; capsule intact, no tumor on ovarian surface; no malignant cells in ascites or peritoneal washings[1] (Figure 30.2)
T1b	IB	Tumor limited to both ovaries; capsule intact, no tumor on ovarian surface; no malignant cells in ascites or peritoneal washings[1] (Figure 30.3)
T1c	IC	Tumor limited to one or both ovaries with any of the following: capsule ruptured, tumor on ovarian surface, malignant cells in ascites or peritoneal washings (Figure 30.4)
T2	II	Tumor involves one or both ovaries with pelvic extension
T2a	IIA	Extension and/or implants on uterus and/or tube(s); no malignant cells in ascites or peritoneal washings (Figure 30.5)
T2b	IIB	Extension to and/or implants on other pelvic tissues; no malignant cells in ascites or peritoneal washings (Figure 30.6)

TNM: **T1a**
FIGO: IA

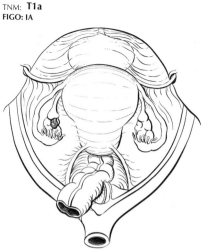

FIGURE 30.2. T1a is tumor limited to one ovary; capsule intact, no tumor on ovarian surface, and no malignant cells in ascites or peritoneal washings.[1]

TNM: **T1b**
FIGO: IB

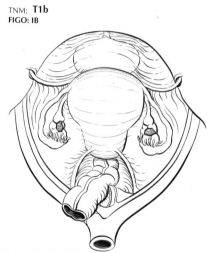

FIGURE 30.3. T1b is tumor limited to both ovaries; capsule intact, no tumor on ovarian surface. No malignant cells in ascites or peritoneal washings.[1]

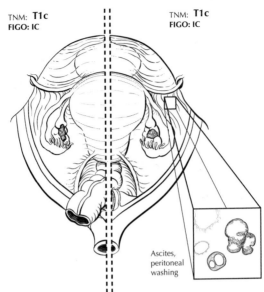

Ascites,
peritoneal
washing

FIGURE 30.4. Two views of T1c, defined as tumor limited to one or both ovaries with any of the following: capsule ruptured, tumor on ovarian surface (left side of dotted line), malignant cells in ascites or peritoneal washings (right side of dotted line).

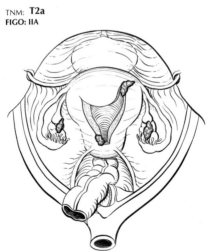

FIGURE 30.5. T2 is tumor involving one or both ovaries with pelvic extension. T2a involves extension and/or implants on uterus (shown) and/or tube(s) without any malignant cells in ascites or peritoneal washings.

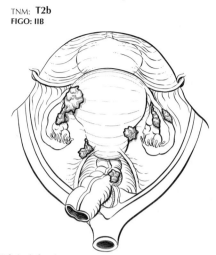

FIGURE 30.6. T2b is defined as tumor extension to and/or implants on other pelvic tissues. No malignant cells in ascites or peritoneal washings.

| T2c | IIC | Pelvic extension and/or implants (T2a or T2b) with malignant cells in ascites or peritoneal washings (Figure 30.7) |
| T3 | III | Tumor involves one or both ovaries with microscopically confirmed peritoneal metastasis outside the pelvis[2] (Figures 30.8, 30.9) |

TNM: **T2c**
FIGO: IIC

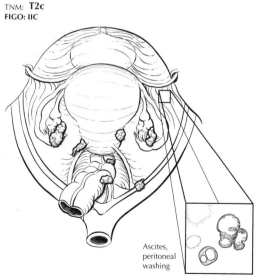

Ascites, peritoneal washing

FIGURE 30.7. T2c is defined as tumor with pelvic extension and/or implants (T2a or T2b) and with malignant cells in ascites or peritoneal washings.

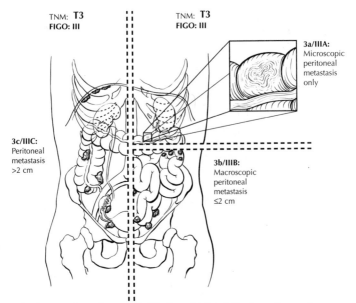

FIGURE 30.8. Three views of T3: T3a (top right) is defined as microscopic peritoneal metastasis beyond pelvis (no macroscopic tumor)[2]; T3b (bottom right) is defined as macroscopic peritoneal metastasis beyond pelvis 2 cm or less in greatest dimension[2]; T3c (left side) is defined as peritoneal metastasis beyond pelvis more than 2 cm in greatest dimension and/or regional lymph node metastasis.

| T3a | IIIA | Microscopic peritoneal metastasis beyond pelvis (no macroscopic tumor)[2] (Figure 30.8) |
| T3b | IIIB | Macroscopic peritoneal metastasis beyond pelvis 2 cm or less in greatest dimension[2] (Figure 30.8) |

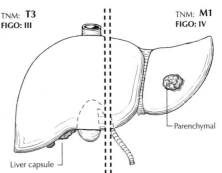

FIGURE 30.9. Liver capsule metastasis classified as T3/Stage III. Liver parenchymal metastasis classified as M1/Stage IV.

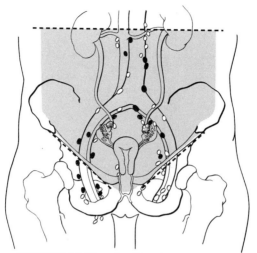

30

FIGURE 30.10. N1: regional lymph node metastasis.

T3c   IIIC   Peritoneal metastasis beyond pelvis more than 2 cm in great-
                est dimension and/or regional lymph node metastasis[2]
                (Figure 30.8)

Regional Lymph Nodes (N)

NX   Regional lymph nodes cannot be assessed
N0   No regional lymph node metastasis
N1   IIIC   Regional lymph node metastasis (Figure 30.10)

Distant Metastasis (M)

MX   Distant metastasis cannot be assessed
M0   No distant metastasis
M1   IV   Distant metastasis (excludes peritoneal metastasis)[2] (Figure 30.9)

STAGE GROUPING (AJCC/UICC/FIGO)

I	T1	N0	M0
IA	T1a	N0	M0
IB	T1b	N0	M0
IC	T1c	N0	M0
II	T2	N0	M0
IIA	T2a	N0	M0
IIB	T2b	N0	M0
IIC	T2c	N0	M0
III	T3	N0	M0
IIIA	T3a	N0	M0

IIIB	T3b	N0	M0
IIIC	T3c	N0	M0
	Any T	N1	M0
IV	Any T	Any N	M1

NOTES

1. The presence of nonmalignant ascites is not classified. The presence of ascites does not affect staging unless malignant cells are present.
2. Liver capsule metastasis T3/III, liver parenchymal metastasis M1/Stage IV. Pleural effusion must have positive cytology for M1/Stage IV.

...

Fallopian Tube

C57.0   Fallopian tube

SUMMARY OF CHANGES

• The definitions of TNM and Stage Grouping for this chapter have not changed from the Fifth Edition.

ANATOMY

Primary Site. The fallopian tube extends from the posterior superior aspect of the uterine fundus laterally and anteriorly to the ovary. Its length is approximately 10 cm. The medial end arises in the cornual portion of the uterine cavity, and the lateral end opens to the peritoneal cavity.

Carcinoma of the fallopian tube is almost always an adenocarcinoma arising from an *in situ* lesion of the tubal mucosa. It invades locally into the muscular wall of the tube and then into the peritubal soft tissue or adjacent organs such as the uterus or ovary, or through the serosa of the tube into the peritoneal cavity. Metastatic tumor implants can be found throughout the peritoneal cavity. The tumor may obstruct the tubal lumen and present as a ruptured or unruptured hydrosalpinx or hematosalpinx.

Regional Nodes. Carcinoma of the fallopian tube can also metastasize to the regional lymph nodes (see Figure 30.1), which include:

Common iliac
Internal iliac (hypogastric)
Obturator
Presacral
Para-aortic
Inguinal
Pelvic lymph nodes, NOS

Adequate evaluation of the regional lymph nodes usually includes aortic and pelvic nodes.

Distant Metastases. Surface implants within the pelvic cavity and the abdominal cavity are common, but these are classified as T2 and T3 disease, respectively. Parenchymal liver metastases and extraperitoneal sites, including lung and skeletal metastases, are M1 (see Figure 30.9).

DEFINITIONS

Primary Tumor (T)

TNM	FIGO
Categories	*Stages*
TX	Primary tumor cannot be assessed
T0	No evidence of primary tumor

TNM: **T1a**
FIGO: **IA**

FIGURE 31.1. T1a is tumor limited to one fallopian tube, without penetrating the serosal surface; no ascites.

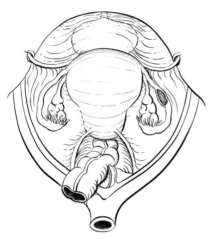

Tis	0	Carcinoma *in situ* (limited to tubal mucosa)
T1	I	Tumor limited to the fallopian tube(s)
T1a	IA	Tumor limited to one tube, without penetrating the serosal surface; no ascites (Figure 31.1)
T1b	IB	Tumor limited to both tubes, without penetrating the serosal surface; no ascites (Figure 31.2)

TNM: **T1b**
FIGO: **IB**

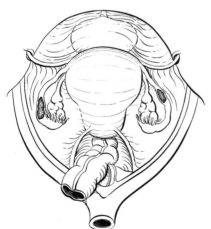

FIGURE 31.2. T1b is tumor limited to both tubes, without penetrating the serosal surface; no ascites.

T1c	IC	Tumor limited to one or both tubes with extension onto or through the tubal serosa, or with malignant cells in ascites or peritoneal washings (Figure 31.3)
T2	II	Tumor involves one or both fallopian tubes with pelvic extension
T2a	IIA	Extension and/or metastasis to the uterus and/or ovaries (Figure 31.4)
T2b	IIB	Extension to other pelvic structures (Figure 31.5)
T2c	IIC	Pelvic extension with malignant cells in ascites or peritoneal washings (Figure 31.6)
T3	III	Tumor involves one or both fallopian tubes, with peritoneal implants outside the pelvis
T3a	IIIA	Microscopic peritoneal metastasis outside the pelvis
T3b	IIIB	Macroscopic peritoneal metastasis outside the pelvis 2 cm or less in greatest dimension
T3c	IIIC	Peritoneal metastasis more than 2 cm in diameter

Regional Lymph Nodes (N)

NX		Regional lymph nodes cannot be assessed
N0		No regional lymph node metastasis
N1	IIIC	Regional lymph node metastasis

Distant Metastasis (M)

MX		Distant metastasis cannot be assessed
M0		No distant metastasis
M1	IV	Distant metastasis (excludes metastasis within the peritoneal cavity)

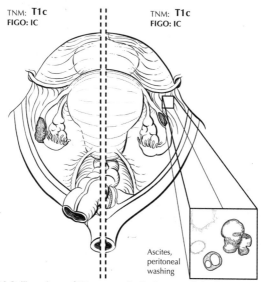

TNM: **T1c**
FIGO: **IC**

TNM: **T1c**
FIGO: **IC**

Ascites, peritoneal washing

FIGURE 31.3. Two views of T1c: tumor limited to one (left of dotted line) or both tubes with extension onto or through the tubal serosa, or with malignant cells in ascites or peritoneal washings (right of the dotted line).

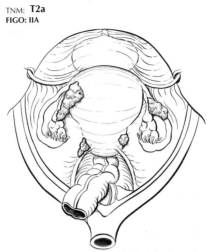

TNM: **T2a**
FIGO: IIA

FIGURE 31.4. T2a is tumor involving one or both fallopian tubes with pelvic extension and/or metastasis to the uterus (shown) and/or ovaries.

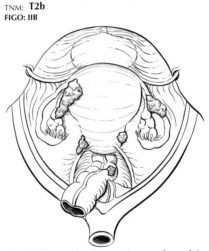

TNM: **T2b**
FIGO: IIB

FIGURE 31.5. T2b is tumor with extension to other pelvic structures.

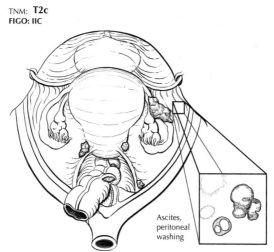

TNM: **T2c**
FIGO: **IIC**

Ascites,
peritoneal
washing

31

FIGURE 31.6. T2c is pelvic extension with malignant cells in ascites or peritoneal washings.

STAGE GROUPING (AJCC/UICC/FIGO)

0	Tis	N0	M0
I	T1	N0	M0
IA	T1a	N0	M0
IB	T1b	N0	M0
IC	T1c	N0	M0
II	T2	N0	M0
IIA	T2a	N0	M0
IIB	T2b	N0	M0
IIC	T2c	N0	M0
III	T3	N0	M0
IIIA	T3a	N0	M0
IIIB	T3b	N0	M0
IIIC	T3c	N0	M0
	Any T	N1	M0
IV	Any T	Any N	M1

Gestational Trophoblastic Tumors

C58.9   Placenta

SUMMARY OF CHANGES

• Gestational trophoblastic tumors are effectively treated with chemotherapy even when widely metastatic so that traditional anatomic staging parameters do not adequately provide different diagnostic categories. For this reason, although the anatomic categories are preserved, a scoring system of other nonanatomic risk factors has been added. This risk factor score provides the basis for substaging patients into A (low risk, score of 7 or less) or B (high risk, score of 8 or greater).

• The "Risk Factors" portion of the stage grouping has been revised to reflect the new scoring system.

INTRODUCTION

Gestational trophoblastic tumors are uncommon (1 in 1,000 pregnancies) malignancies that arise from the placenta. Usually as a result of a genetic accident in the developing egg, the maternal chromosomes are lost, and the paternal chromosomes duplicate (46xxx). The resulting tumor is known as a *complete* hydatidiform mole: there are no fetal parts; the tumor is composed of dilated, avascular, "grape-like" vesicles that may grow as large as, or larger than, the normal pregnancy it replaces. There is obviously no heartbeat detected, and the patient may have vaginal bleeding similar to a miscarriage. Many times, the diagnosis is not made until a dilatation and curettage is done and the tissue is examined pathologically. In some patients, fetal parts will be found in association with mild proliferative trophoblastic (placental) tissues. Such patients have a *partial* hydatidiform mole, which has a 69xxx or 69xxy chromosomal complement resulting from twice the normal number of paternal chromosomes. Both of these tumors usually follow a benign course, resolving completely after evacuation by the dilatation and suction or curettage, but approximately 20% of complete moles and 5% of partial moles persist locally or metastasize and thus require chemotherapy.

Much less frequently (about 1 in 20,000 pregnancies in the United States), a highly malignant, rapidly growing metastatic form of gestational trophoblastic disease called choriocarcinoma is encountered. This solid, anaplastic, avascular, and aggressively proliferative tumor is easily recognized microscopically and may present with symptoms of vaginal bleeding (as with a hydatidiform mole). However, metastatic lesions may be the first sign of this lesion, which can follow any pregnancy event, including an incomplete abortion or a full-term pregnancy.

The trophoblastic tissue that makes up these tumors produces a serum tumor marker, beta-human chorionic gonadotrophin (β-hCG), which is very helpful in the diagnosis and monitoring of therapy in these patients. Gestational

---

trophoblastic tumors are very responsive to chemotherapy, with cure rates approaching 100%.

ANATOMY

Because of the responsiveness of this tumor to treatment and the accuracy of the serum marker hCG in reflecting the status of disease, the traditional anatomic staging system used in most solid tumors has little prognostic significance. Trophoblastic tumors not associated with pregnancy (ovarian teratomas) are not included in this classification.

Primary Site. By definition, gestational trophoblastic tumors arise from placental tissue in the uterus. Although most of these tumors are noninvasive and are removed by dilatation and suction evacuation, local invasion of the myometrium can occur. When this is diagnosed on a hysterectomy specimen (rarely done these days), it may be reported as an *invasive* hydatidiform mole.

Regional Lymph Nodes. Nodal involvement in gestational trophoblastic tumors is rare but has a very poor prognosis when diagnosed. There is no regional designation in the staging of these tumors. Nodal metastases should be classified as metastatic (M1) disease.

Metastatic Sites. This is a highly vascular tumor that results in frequent, widespread metastases when these lesions become malignant. The cervix and vagina are common pelvic sites of metastases (T2), and the lungs are often involved by distant metastases (M1a). Other, less frequently encountered metastatic sites include kidney, gastrointestinal tract, and spleen (M1b). The liver and brain are occasionally involved and may harbor metastatic sites that are difficult to treat with chemotherapy.

DEFINITIONS

Primary Tumor (T)[1]

TNM*	FIGO	
Categories	Stages	
TX		Primary tumor cannot be assessed
T0		No evidence of primary tumor
T1	I	Disease limited to uterus (Figure 32.1)
T2	II	Disease outside of uterus but limited to genital structures (ovary, tube, vagina, broad ligaments) (Figure 32.2)

Distant Metastasis (M)

MX		Metastasis cannot be assessed
M0		No distant metastasis
M1		Distant metastasis
M1a	III	Lung metastasis (Figure 32.3)
M1b	IV	All other distant metastasis (Figure 32.4)

Note: There is no regional nodal staging for this tumor.

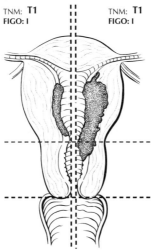

FIGURE 32.1. Two views of T1 (disease confined to the uterus): tumor confined to endometrium (left side of dotted line) and tumor with invasion of myometrium and cervix (right side of dotted line).

32

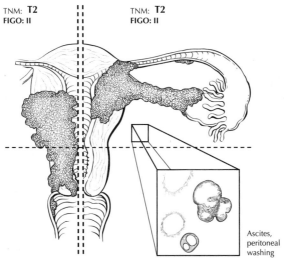

FIGURE 32.2. Two views of T2 (disease outside of the uterus but limited to genital structures): involvement of the vagina (left side of the dotted line), fallopian tube and ovary as well as the presence of malignant ascites (right side of the dotted line).

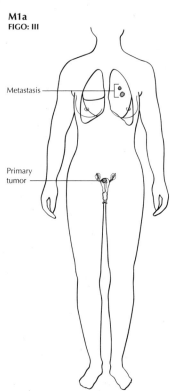

M1a
FIGO: III

Metastasis

Primary
tumor

FIGURE 32.3. M1a is defined as metastatic disease to the lung.

STAGE GROUPING[2]

	Stage T	M	Risk Factors
I	T1	M0	Unknown
IA	T1	M0	Low risk
IB	T1	M0	High risk
II	T2	M0	Unknown
IIA	T2	M0	Low risk
IIB	T2	M0	High risk
III	Any T	M1a	Unknown
IIIA	Any T	M1a	Low risk
IIIB	Any T	M1a	High risk
IV	Any T	M1b	Unknown
IVA	Any T	M1b	Low risk
IVB	Any T	M1b	High risk

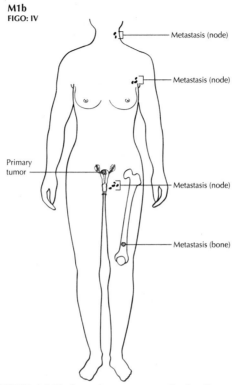

M1b
FIGO: IV

Metastasis (node)

Metastasis (node)

Primary tumor

Metastasis (node)

Metastasis (bone)

FIGURE 32.4. M1b disease is metastases to all other distant sites.

TABLE 32.1 Prognostic Indicators Scoring Index

	Risk Score			
Prognostic Factor	*0*	*1*	*2*	*4*
Age	<40	>40		
Antecedent pregnancy	H. mole	Abortion	Term pregnancy	
Interval months from index pregnancy	<4	4–<7	7–12	>12
Pretreatment hCG (IU/ml)	<10³	≥10³–<10⁴	10⁴–<10⁵	≥10⁵
Largest tumor size including uterus	<3 cm	3–<5 cm	≥5 cm	
Site of metastases	Lung	Spleen, kidney	Gastrointestinal tract	Brain, liver
Number of metastases identified		1–4	5–8	>8
Previous failed chemotherapy			Single drug	Two or more drugs

Total Score
Low risk is a score of 7 or less. *High risk* is a score of 8 or greater.

NOTES

1. See Table 32.1, prognostic indicator section for substage definitions.
2. See Table 32.1, prognostic indicators for substage grouping.

PART VIII
Genitourinary Sites

Penis

(Melanomas are not included.)

C60.0	Prepuce	C60.8	Overlapping lesion of	C60.9	Penis, NOS
C60.1	Glans penis		penis		
C60.2	Body of penis				

SUMMARY OF CHANGES

• The definitions of TNM and the Stage Grouping for this chapter have not changed from the Fifth Edition.

INTRODUCTION

Cancers of the penis are rare in the United States, although the incidence varies in different countries of the world. Most are squamous cell carcinomas that arise in the skin or on the glans penis. Prognosis is favorable provided that the lymph nodes are not involved. Melanomas can also occur. The staging classification, however, applies to carcinomas. Melanomas are staged in Chapter 24. Some cancers of the penis may be described as verrucous. Similarly, basaloid tumors are recognized as a subtype of squamous carcinoma. An *in situ* lesion is also included and by definition should be coded as an *in situ* carcinoma of the penis.

ANATOMY

Primary Site. The penis is composed of three cylindrical masses of cavernous tissue bound together by fibrous tissue. Two masses are lateral and are known as the corpora cavernosa penis. The corpus spongiosum penis is a median mass and contains the greater part of the urethra. The penis is attached to the front and the sides of the pubic arch. The skin covering the penis is thin and loosely connected with the deeper parts of the organ. The skin at the root of the penis is continuous with that over the scrotum and perineum. Distally, the skin becomes folded upon itself to form the prepuce, or foreskin. Anatomical sites are illustrated in Figure 33.1. Circumcision has been associated with a decreased incidence of cancer of the penis.

Regional Lymph Nodes. The regional lymph nodes are:

Single superficial inguinal (femoral)
Multiple or bilateral superficial inguinal (femoral)
Deep inguinal: Rosenmuller's or Cloquet's node
External iliac
Internal iliac (hypogastric)
Pelvic nodes, NOS

Metastatic Sites. Lung, liver, and bone are most often involved.

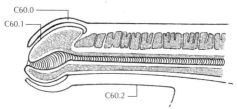

FIGURE 33.1. Anatomic sites and subsites of the penis.

DEFINITIONS

Primary Tumor (T)

TX   Primary tumor cannot be assessed
T0   No evidence of primary tumor
Tis   Carcinoma *in situ*
Ta   Noninvasive verrucous carcinoma (Figure 33.2)
T1   Tumor invades subepithelial connective tissue (Figure 33.3)
T2   Tumor invades corpus spongiosum or cavernosum (Figure 33.4)
T3   Tumor invades urethra or prostate (Figures 33.5A, B)
T4   Tumor invades other adjacent structures (Figures 33.6, 33.7)

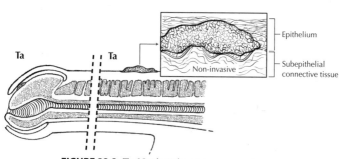

FIGURE 33.2. Ta: Noninvasive verrucous carcinoma.

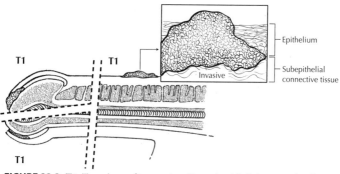

FIGURE 33.3. T1: Two views of tumor invading subepithelial connective tissue.

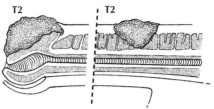

FIGURE 33.4. T2: Two views of tumor invading corpus spongiosum or cavernosum.

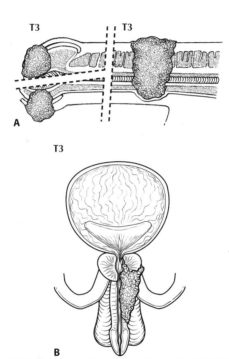

FIGURE 33.5. A. T3: Two views of tumor invading urethra. **B.** T3: Tumor invades prostate.

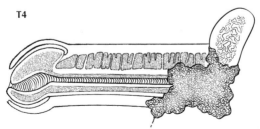

FIGURE 33.6. T4: Tumor invades other adjacent structures.

T4

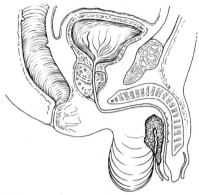

FIGURE 33.7. T4: Tumor invades other adjacent structures.

Regional Lymph Nodes (N)

NX   Regional lymph nodes cannot be assessed
N0   No regional lymph node metastasis
N1   Metastasis in a single superficial inguinal lymph node (Figure 33.8)
N2   Metastasis in multiple or bilateral superficial inguinal lymph nodes (Figures 33.9A, B)
N3   Metastasis in deep inguinal or pelvic lymph node(s), unilateral or bilateral (Figures 33.10A–C)

Distant Metastasis (M)

MX   Distant metastasis cannot be assessed
M0   No distant metastasis
M1   Distant metastasis

N1

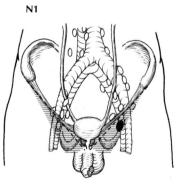

FIGURE 33.8. N1: Metastasis in a single superficial inguinal lymph node.

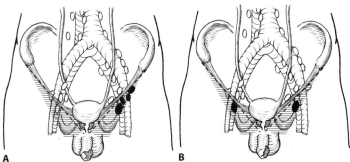

FIGURE 33.9. A. N2: Metastasis in multiple, as shown above, or bilateral superficial inguinal lymph nodes. **B.** N2: Metastasis in bilateral superficial inguinal nodes.

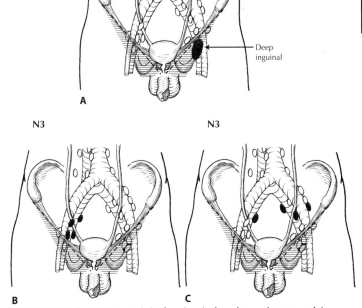

FIGURE 33.10. A. N3: Metastasis in deep inguinal, as shown above, or pelvic lymph node(s), unilateral or bilateral. **B.** N3: Metastasis in unilateral pelvic lymph node(s). **C.** N3: Metastasis in bilateral pelvic lymph node(s).

STAGE GROUPING

0	Tis	N0	M0
	Ta	N0	M0
I	T1	N0	M0
II	T1	N1	M0
	T2	N0	M0
	T2	N1	M0
III	T1	N2	M0
	T2	N2	M0
	T3	N0	M0
	T3	N1	M0
	T3	N2	M0
IV	T4	Any N	M0
	Any T	N3	M0
	Any T	Any N	M1

Prostate

(Sarcomas and transitional cell carcinomas are not included.)

C61.9   Prostate gland

SUMMARY OF CHANGES

- T2 lesions have been divided to include T2a, T2b, and T2c once again. These are the same subcategories found in the Fourth Edition of the AJCC Manual.

- Gleason score is emphasized as the grading system of choice and using the terms *well differentiated, moderately differentiated,* and *poorly differentiated* for grading is not recommended.

INTRODUCTION

Prostate cancer is the most common cancer in men, with increasing incidence in older age groups. Prostate cancer has a tendency to metastasize to bone. Earlier detection is possible with a blood test, prostate-specific antigen (PSA), and diagnosis is generally made using transrectal ultrasound (TRUS) guided biopsy.

ANATOMY

Primary Site. Anatomy of the prostate is illustrated in Figure 34.1. Adenocarcinoma of the prostate frequently arises within the peripheral zone of the gland, where it may be amenable to detection by digital rectal examination (DRE). A less common site of origin is the anteromedial prostate, the transition zone, which is remote from the rectal surface and is the site of origin of benign nodular hyperplasia. The central zone, which makes up most of the base of the prostate, seldom gives rise to cancer but is often invaded by the spread of large cancers. Pathologically, cancers of the prostate are often multifocal.

There is agreement that the incidence of both clinical and latent carcinoma increases with age. However, this cancer is rarely diagnosed clinically in men under 40 years of age. There are substantial limitations in the ability of both DRE and TRUS to define precisely the size or local extent of disease; DRE is currently the most common modality used to define the local stage. Heterogeneity within the T1c category resulting from inherent limitations of either DRE or imaging to quantify the cancer may be balanced by the inclusion of other prognostic factors, such as histologic grade, PSA level, and possibly extent of cancer on needle biopsies that contain cancer. Diagnosis of clinically suspicious areas of the prostate can be confirmed histologically by needle biopsy. Less commonly, prostate cancer may be diagnosed by inspection of the resected tissue from a transurethral resection of the prostate (TURP) for obstructive voiding symptoms.

The histologic grade of the prostate cancer is important for prognosis. The histopathologic grading of these tumors can be complex because of the

---

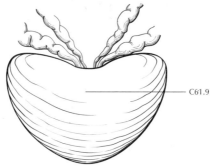

FIGURE 34.1. Anatomy of the prostate.

morphologic heterogeneity so often encountered in surgical specimens. Either a histologic or a pattern type of grading method can be used. The Gleason score for assessing the histologic pattern of prostate cancer is preferred.

Regional Lymph Nodes. The regional lymph nodes are the nodes of the true pelvis, which essentially are the pelvic nodes below the bifurcation of the common iliac arteries (Figure 34.2). They include the following groups:

Pelvic NOS
Hypogastric
Obturator
Iliac (internal, external, or NOS)
Sacral (lateral, presacral, promontory [Gerota's], or NOS)

Laterality does not affect the "N" classification.

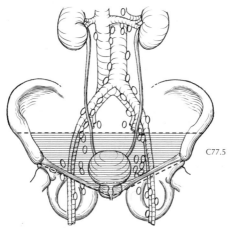

FIGURE 34.2. Shaded area represents regional distribution of lymph nodes. Nonshaded area indicates nodes outside of regional distribution.

Distant Lymph Nodes. Distant lymph nodes lie outside the confines of the true pelvis. They can be imaged using ultrasound, computed tomography, magnetic resonance imaging, or lymphangiography. Although enlarged lymph nodes can occasionally be visualized, because of a stage migration associated with PSA screening, very few patients will be found to have nodal disease, so false-positive and false-negative results are common when imaging tests are employed. In lieu of imaging, risk tables are generally used to determine individual patient risk of nodal involvement. Involvement of distant lymph nodes is classified as M1a. The distant lymph nodes include:

Aortic (para-aortic lumbar)
Common iliac
Inguinal, deep
Superficial inguinal (femoral)
Supraclavicular
Cervical
Scalene
Retroperitoneal, NOS

The significance of regional lymph node metastasis, pN, in staging prostate cancer lies in the presence of metastatic foci within the lymph nodes.

Metastatic Sites. Osteoblastic metastases are the most common non-nodal site of prostate cancer metastasis. In addition, this tumor frequently spreads to distant lymph nodes. Lung and liver metastases are usually identified late in the course of the disease.

DEFINITIONS

Primary Tumor (T)

Clinical
TX   Primary tumor cannot be assessed
T0   No evidence of primary tumor
T1   Clinically inapparent tumor neither palpable nor visible by imaging
T1a   Tumor incidental histologic finding in 5% or less of tissue resected
      (Figure 34.3)

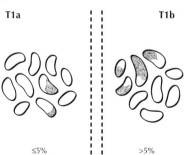

FIGURE 34.3. T1a (left) shows tumor incidental histologic finding in 5% or less of tissue resected. T1b (right) shows tumor incidental histologic finding in more than 5% of tissue resected.

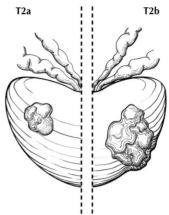

FIGURE 34.4. T2a (left) shows tumor involving one-half of one lobe or less whereas T2b (right) shows tumor involving more than one-half of one lobe but not both lobes.

T1b   Tumor incidental histologic finding in more than 5% of tissue resected (Figure 34.3)

T1c   Tumor identified by needle biopsy (e.g., because of elevated PSA)

T2   Tumor confined within prostate[1]

T2a   Tumor involves one-half of one lobe or less (Figure 34.4)

T2b   Tumor involves more than one-half of one lobe but not both lobes (Figure 34.4)

T2c   Tumor involves both lobes (Figure 34.5)

T3   Tumor extends through the prostate capsule[2]

T3a   Extracapsular extension (unilateral or bilateral) (Figures 34.6A, B)

T3b   Tumor invades seminal vesicle(s) (Figure 34.7)

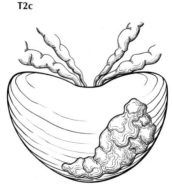

FIGURE 34.5. T2c tumor involving both lobes

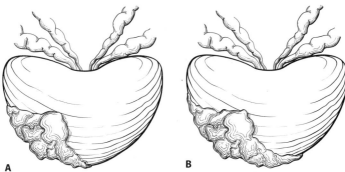

T3a   **T3a**

A   **B**

FIGURE 34.6. A,B. T3a is defined as a tumor with unilateral extracapsular extension, as shown in **A**, or with bilateral extracapsular extension, as shown in **B**.

T4   Tumor is fixed or invades adjacent structures other than seminal vesicles: bladder neck, external sphincter, rectum, levator muscles, and/or pelvic wall (Figures 34.8A, B)

Pathologic (pT)[3]

pT2   Organ confined
pT2a   Unilateral, one-half of one lobe or less
pT2b   Unilateral, involving more than one-half of lobe but not both lobes
pT2c   Bilateral disease
pT3   Extraprostatic extension
pT3a   Extraprostatic extension[4]
pT3b   Seminal vesicle invasion
pT4   Invasion of bladder, rectum

34

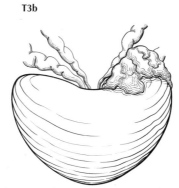

T3b

FIGURE 34.7. T3b tumor invading seminal vesicle(s).

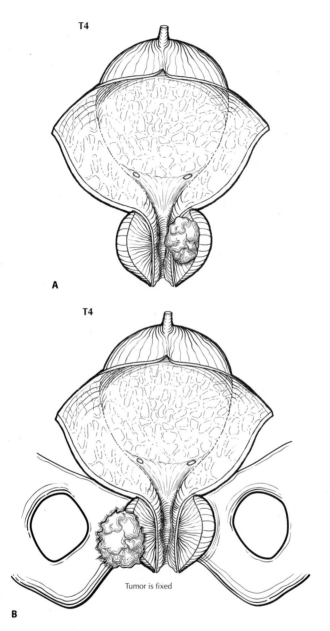

FIGURE 34.8. A. T4 tumor invading adjacent structures other than seminal vesicles such as bladder neck, as shown here, external sphincter, rectum, levator muscles, and/or pelvic wall or tumor is fixed. **B.** T4 showing tumor fixed to adjacent structures.

Regional Lymph Nodes (N)

Clinical

NX   Regional lymph nodes were not assessed

N0   No regional lymph node metastasis

N1   Metastasis in regional lymph node(s) (Figures 34.9A, B)

N1

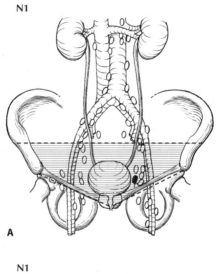

A

N1

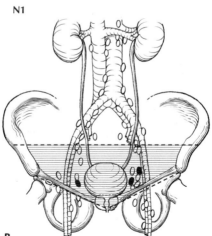

B

FIGURE 34.9. A. N1 metastasis in regional lymph nodes, here shown unilaterally. **B.** N1 metastasis in regional lymph nodes, here shown bilaterally.

Regional Lymph Nodes (N)

Pathologic
pNX   Regional nodes not sampled
pN0   No positive regional nodes
pN1   Metastases in regional node(s)

Distant Metastasis (M)[5]

MX   Distant metastasis cannot be assessed (not evaluated by any modality)
M0   No distant metastasis
M1   Distant metastasis
M1a   Nonregional lymph node(s)
M1b   Bone(s)
M1c   Other site(s) with or without bone disease

STAGE GROUPING

I	T1a	N0	M0	G1
II	T1a	N0	M0	G2,3–4
	T1b	N0	M0	Any G
	T1c	N0	M0	Any G
	T1	N0	M0	Any G
	T2	N0	M0	Any G
III	T3	N0	M0	Any G
IV	T4	N0	M0	Any G
	Any T	N1	M0	Any G
	Any T	Any N	M1	Any G

HISTOLOGIC GRADE (G)

Gleason score is considered to be the optimal method of grading, because this method takes into account the inherent heterogeneity of prostate cancer, and because it has been clearly shown that this method is of great prognostic value. A primary and secondary pattern (the range of each is 1–5) are assigned and then summed to yield a total score. Scores of 2–10 are thus possible. (If a single focus of disease is seen, it should be reported as both scores. For example, if a single focus of Gleason 3 disease is seen, it is reported as 3 + 3).

GX   Grade cannot be assessed
G1   Well differentiated (slight anaplasia) (Gleason 2–4)
G2   Moderately differentiated (moderate anaplasia) (Gleason 5–6)
G3–4   Poorly differentiated/undifferentiated (marked anaplasia) (Gleason 7–10)

NOTES

1. Tumor found in one or both lobes by needle biopsy, but not palpable or reliably visible by imaging, is classified as T1c.
2. Invasion into the prostatic apex or into (but not beyond) the prostatic capsule is classified not as T3, but as T2.
3. There is no pathologic T1 classification.

4. Positive surgical margin should be indicated by an R1 descriptor (residual microscopic disease).
5. When more than one site of metastasis is present, the most advanced category is used. pM1c is most advanced.

35

Testis

C62.0   Undescended testis   C62.1   Descended testis   C62.9   Testis, NOS

SUMMARY OF CHANGES

• The definitions of TNM and the Stage Grouping for this chapter have not changed from the Fifth Edition.

INTRODUCTION

Cancers of the testis are usually found in young adults and account for less than 1% of all malignancies in males. However, during the twentieth century, the incidence has more than doubled. Cryptorchidism is a predisposing condition, and other associations include atypical germ cells and multiple atypical nevi. Germ cell tumors of the testis are categorized into two main histologic types: seminomas and non-seminomas. The latter group is composed of either individual or combinations of histologic subtypes, including embryonal carcinoma, teratoma, choriocarcinoma, and yolk sac tumor. The presence of serum markers, including alpha-fetoprotein (AFP), human chorionic gonadotropin (hCG), and lactate dehydrogenase (LDH), is frequent in this disease. Staging and prognostication are based on the determination of the extent of disease and assessment of serum tumor markers. Cancer of the testis is highly curable, even in cases with advanced, metastatic disease.

ANATOMY

Primary Site. The anatomy of the testes is illustrated in Figure 35.1. The testes are composed of convoluted seminiferous tubules with a stroma containing functional endocrine interstitial cells. Both are encased in a dense capsule, the tunica albuginea, with fibrous septa extending into the testes and separating them into lobules. The tubules converge and exit at the mediastinum of the testis into the rete testis and efferent ducts, which join a single duct. This duct—the epididymis—coils outside the upper and lower poles of the testicle and then joins the vas deferens, a muscular conduit that accompanies the vessels and lymphatic channels of the spermatic cord. The major route for local extension of cancer is through the lymphatic channels. The tumor emerges from the mediastinum of the testis and courses through the spermatic cord. Occasionally, the epididymis is invaded early, and then the external iliac nodes may become involved. If there has been previous scrotal or inguinal surgery or if invasion of the scrotal wall is found (though this is rare), then the lymphatic spread may be to inguinal nodes.

Regional Lymph Nodes. The following nodes are considered regional (Figure 35.2):

Interaortocaval
Para-aortic (periaortic)

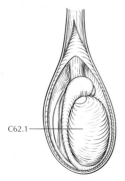

FIGURE 35.1. Anatomy of the testis.

C62.1

Paracaval
Preaortic
Precaval
Retroaortic
Retrocaval

The intrapelvic, external iliac, and inguinal nodes are considered regional only after scrotal or inguinal surgery prior to the presentation of the testis tumor.

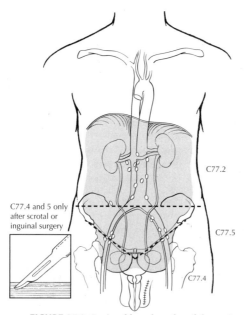

C77.2

C77.4 and 5 only
after scrotal or
inguinal surgery

C77.5

C77.4

FIGURE 35.2. Regional lymph nodes of the testis.

All nodes outside the regional nodes are distant. Nodes along the spermatic vein are considered regional.

Metastatic Site. Distant spread of testicular tumors occurs most commonly to the lymph nodes, followed by metastases to the lung, liver, bone, and other visceral sites. Stage is dependent on the extent of disease and on the determination of serum tumor markers. Extent of disease includes assessment for involvement and size of regional lymph nodes, evidence of disease in nonregional lymph nodes, and metastases to pulmonary and non-pulmonary visceral sites. The stage is subdivided on the basis of the presence and degree of elevation of serum tumor markers. Serum tumor markers are measured immediately after orchiectomy and, if elevated, should be measured serially after orchiectomy to determine whether normal decay curves are followed. The physiological half-life of AFP is 5–7 days, and the half-life of HCG is 24–48 hours. The presence of prolonged half-life times implies the presence of residual disease after orchiectomy. It should be noted that in some cases, tumor marker release may occur (for example, in response to chemotherapy or handling of a primary tumor intraoperatively) and may cause artificial elevation of circulating tumor marker levels. The serum level of lactate dehydrogenase (LDH) has prognostic value in patients with metastatic disease and is included for staging.

DEFINITIONS

Primary Tumor (T)[1]

The extent of primary tumor is usually classified after radical orchiectomy, and for this reason, a *pathologic* stage is assigned.

pTX   Primary tumor cannot be assessed (if no radical orchiectomy has been performed, TX is used)
pT0   No evidence of primary tumor (e.g., histologic scar in testis)
pTis   Intratubular germ cell neoplasia (carcinoma *in situ*)
pT1   Tumor limited to the testis and epididymis without vascular/lymphatic invasion; tumor may invade into the tunica albuginea but not the tunica vaginalis (Figure 35.3A)
pT2   Tumor limited to the testis and epididymis with vascular/lymphatic invasion, or tumor extending through the tunica albuginea with involvement of the tunica vaginalis (Figures 35.3A, B)
pT3   Tumor invades the spermatic cord with or without vascular/lymphatic invasion (Figure 35.4)
pT4   Tumor invades the scrotum with or without vascular/lymphatic invasion (Figure 35.5)

Regional Lymph Nodes (N)

Clinical
NX   Regional lymph nodes cannot be assessed
N0   No regional lymph node metastasis
N1   Metastasis with a lymph node mass 2 cm or less in greatest dimension; or multiple lymph nodes, none more than 2 cm in greatest dimension (Figures 35.6A–F)

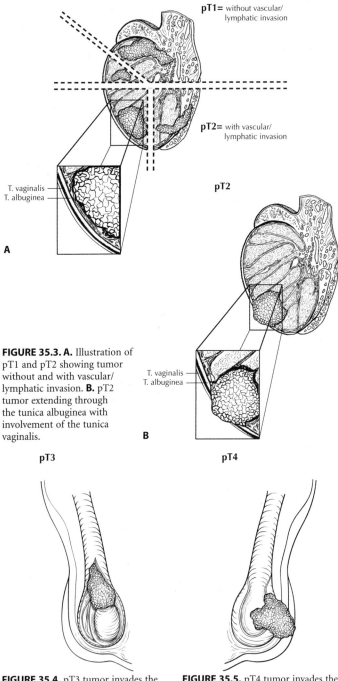

pT1 = without vascular/lymphatic invasion

pT2 = with vascular/lymphatic invasion

pT2

T. vaginalis
T. albuginea

A

T. vaginalis
T. albuginea

B

FIGURE 35.3. A. Illustration of pT1 and pT2 showing tumor without and with vascular/lymphatic invasion. **B.** pT2 tumor extending through the tunica albuginea with involvement of the tunica vaginalis.

pT3

pT4

FIGURE 35.4. pT3 tumor invades the spermatic cord.

FIGURE 35.5. pT4 tumor invades the scrotum.

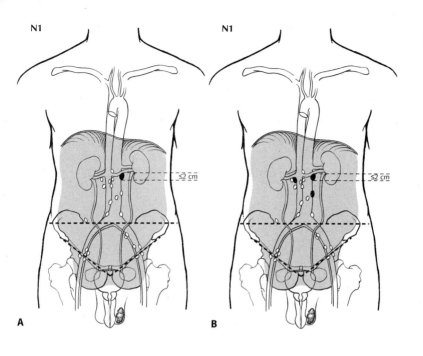

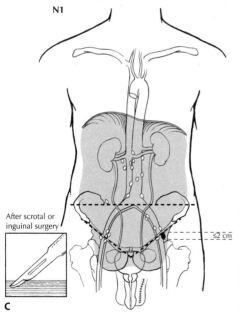

After scrotal or inguinal surgery

FIGURE 35.6. A. N1 is defined as metastasis with a lymph node mass 2 cm or less in greatest dimension. **B.** N1: metastasis in multiple lymph nodes, none more than 2 cm in greatest dimension. **C.** N1: metastasis with a lymph node mass 2 cm or less in greatest dimension, following scrotal or inguinal surgery.

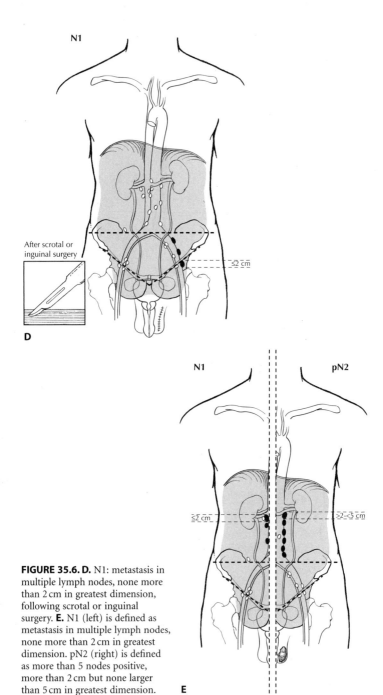

FIGURE 35.6. D. N1: metastasis in multiple lymph nodes, none more than 2 cm in greatest dimension, following scrotal or inguinal surgery. **E.** N1 (left) is defined as metastasis in multiple lymph nodes, none more than 2 cm in greatest dimension. pN2 (right) is defined as more than 5 nodes positive, more than 2 cm but none larger than 5 cm in greatest dimension.

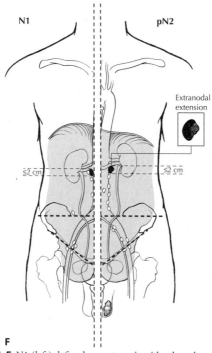

F

FIGURE 35.6. F. N1 (left) defined as metastasis with a lymph node mass 2 cm or less in greatest dimension. pN2 (right) defined as of extranodal extension of tumor.

N2   Metastasis with a lymph node mass more than 2 cm but not more than 5 cm in greatest dimension; or multiple lymph nodes, any one mass greater than 2 cm but not more than 5 cm in greatest dimension (Figures 35.7A–C)

N3   Metastasis with a lymph node mass more than 5 cm in greatest dimension (Figures 35.8A–D)

Regional Lymph Nodes (N)
Pathologic

pNX   Regional lymph nodes cannot be assessed

pN0   No regional lymph node metastasis

pN1   Metastasis with a lymph node mass 2 cm or less in greatest dimension and less than or equal to 5 nodes positive, none more than 2 cm in greatest dimension

pN2   Metastasis with a lymph node mass more than 2 cm but not more than 5 cm in greatest dimension; or more than 5 nodes positive, none more than 5 cm; or evidence of extranodal extension of tumor (Figures 35.6E, F; Figures 35.7A–C)

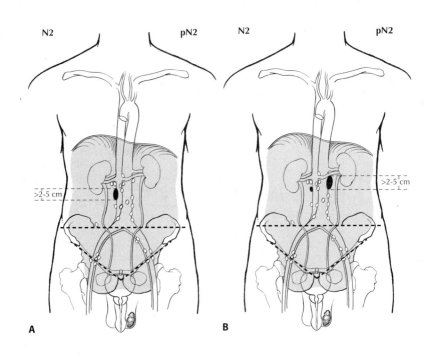

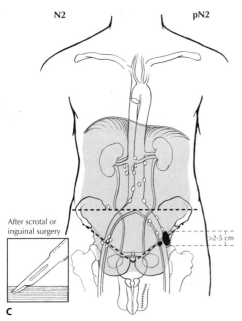

After scrotal or inguinal surgery

FIGURE 35.7. A. N2/pN2: metastasis with a lymph node mass more than 2 cm but not more than 5 cm in greatest dimension. **B.** N2/pN2: metastasis in multiple lymph nodes, any one mass greater than 2 cm but not more than 5 cm in greatest dimension. **C.** N2/pN2: metastasis with a lymph node mass more than 2 cm but not more than 5 cm in greatest dimension, following scrotal or inguinal surgery.

FIGURE 35.8. A. N3/pN3: metastasis with a lymph node mass more than 5 cm in greatest dimension. **B.** N3/pN3 metastasis with a lymph node mass more than 5 cm in greatest dimension, following scrotal or inguinal surgery.

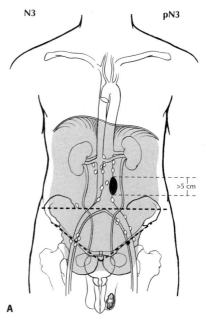

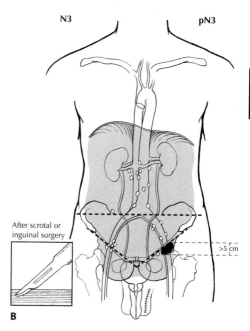

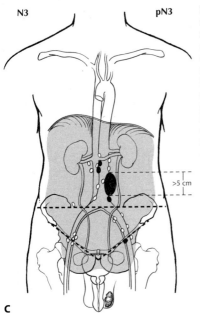

FIGURE 35.8. C. N3/pN3: metastasis with a lymph node mass more than 5 cm in greatest dimension. As illustrated here, multiple nodes are involved with one nodal mass exceeding 5 cm. **D.** N3/pN3: metastasis with a lymph node mass more than 5 cm in greatest dimension. As illustrated here following scrotal or inguinal surgery, multiple nodes are involved with one nodal mass exceeding 5 cm.

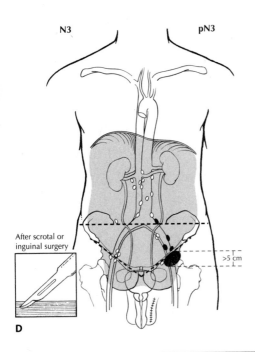

pN3   Metastasis with a lymph node mass more than 5 cm in greatest dimension (Figures 35.8A–D)

Distant Metastasis (M)
MX   Distant metastasis cannot be assessed
M0   No distant metastasis
M1   Distant metastasis
M1a   Nonregional nodal or pulmonary metastasis
M1b   Distant metastasis other than to nonregional lymph nodes and lungs

Serum Tumor Markers (S)
(N indicates the upper limit of normal for the LDH assay.)
SX   Marker studies not available or not performed
S0   Marker study levels within normal limits
S1   LDH <1.5 × N AND
      hCG (mIu/ml) <5,000 AND
      AFP (ng/ml) <1,000
S2   LDH 1.5–10 × N OR
      hCG (mIu/ml) 5,000–50,000 OR
      AFP (ng/ml) 1,000–10,000
S3   LDH >10 × N OR
      hCG (mIu/ml) >50,000 OR
      AFP (ng/ml) >10,000

STAGE GROUPING

0	pTis	N0	M0	S0
I	pT1–4	N0	M0	SX
IA	pT1	N0	M0	S0
IB	pT2	N0	M0	S0
	pT3	N0	M0	S0
	pT4	N0	M0	S0
IS	Any pT/Tx	N0	M0	S1–3
II	Any pT/Tx	N1–3	M0	SX
IIA	Any pT/Tx	N1	M0	S0
	Any pT/Tx	N1	M0	S1
IIB	Any pT/Tx	N2	M0	S0
	Any pT/Tx	N2	M0	S1
IIC	Any pT/Tx	N3	M0	S0
	Any pT/Tx	N3	M0	S1
III	Any pT/Tx	Any N	M1	SX
IIIA	Any pT/Tx	Any N	M1a	S0
	Any pT/Tx	Any N	M1a	SI
IIIB	Any pT/Tx	N1–3	M0	S2
	Any pT/Tx	Any N	M1a	S2
IIIC	Any pT/Tx	N1–3	M0	S3
	Any pT/Tx	Any N	M1a	S3
	Any pT/Tx	Any N	M1b	Any S

35

NOTE

1. Except for pTis and pT4, extent of primary tumor is classified by radical orchiectomy. TX may be used for other categories in the absence of radical orchiectomy.

Kidney

C64.9   Kidney

INTRODUCTION

Cancers of the kidney are relatively rare, accounting for less than 3% of all malignancies. Nearly all malignant tumors are carcinomas arising from the renal tubular epithelium or, less frequently, from the renal pelvis (see Chapter 37). These tumors are more common in males. Pain and hematuria are usually the presenting features, but a majority of kidney tumors are not being detected incidentally in asymptomatic individuals. These carcinomas have a tendency to extend into the renal vein and even into the vena cava. Staging depends on the size of the primary tumor, invasion of the adjacent structures, and vascular extension.

Since publication of the Fifth Edition of the AJCC Cancer Staging Manual, the evidence has become compelling that the T1 category should be subdivided into stages T1a and T1b, the former being tumors of 4 cm or less and the latter being tumors greater than 4 cm to 7 cm. The rationale is twofold: (1) the recurrence of survival difference between the two and (2) the current practice of applying partial nephrectomy for solitary tumors 4 cm or less in diameter. In the case of partial nephrectomy for tumors <4 cm in diameter, evidence suggests that survival outcomes are equivalent to outcomes with radical nephrectomy.

ANATOMY

36

Primary Site. Encased by a fibrous capsule and surrounded by perirenal fat, the kidney consists of the cortex (glomeruli, convoluted tubules) and the medulla (Henle's loops, pyramids of converging tubules). Each papilla opens into the minor calices; these in turn unite in the major calices and drain into the renal pelvis. At the hilus are the pelvis, ureter, and renal artery and vein. Gerota's fascia overlies the psoas and quadratus lumborum. The anatomic sites and subsites of the kidney are illustrated in Figure 36.1.

Regional Lymph Nodes. The regional lymph nodes, illustrated in Figure 36.2, are:

Renal hilar
Paracaval

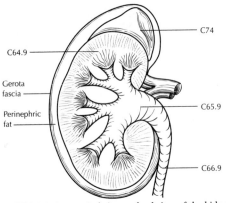

FIGURE 36.1. Anatomical sites and subsites of the kidney.

Aortic (para-aortic, periaortic, lateral aortic)
Retroperitoneal, NOS

Metastatic Sites. Common metastatic sites include bone, liver, lung, brain, and distant lymph nodes.

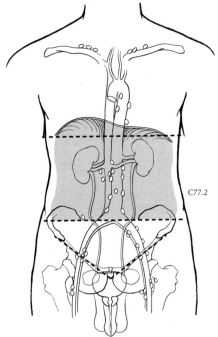

FIGURE 36.2. Regional lymph nodes of the kidney.

T1a

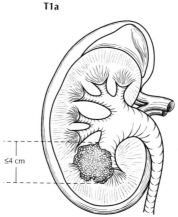

≤4 cm

FIGURE 36.3. T1a: tumor 4 cm or less in greatest dimension, limited to the kidney.

DEFINITIONS

Primary Tumor (T)

TX   Primary tumor cannot be assessed
T0   No evidence of primary tumor
T1   Tumor 7 cm or less in greatest dimension, limited to the kidney
T1a Tumor 4 cm or less in greatest dimension, limited to the kidney (Figure 36.3)
T1b Tumor more than 4 cm but not more than 7 cm in greatest dimension, limited to the kidney (Figure 36.4)

T1b

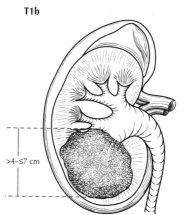

>4–≤7 cm

FIGURE 36.4. T1b: tumor more than 4 cm but not more than 7 cm in greatest dimension, limited to the kidney.

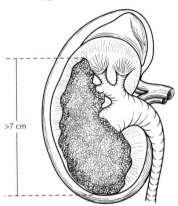

FIGURE 36.5. T2: tumor more than 7 cm in greatest dimension, limited to the kidney.

T2   Tumor more than 7 cm in greatest dimension, limited to the kidney (Figure 36.5)

T3   Tumor extends into major veins or invades adrenal gland or perinephric tissues but not beyond Gerota's fascia

T3a   Tumor directly invades adrenal gland or perirenal and/or renal sinus fat but not beyond Gerota's fascia (Figure 36.6)

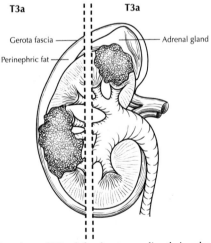

FIGURE 36.6. Two views of T3a, defined as tumor directly invades adrenal gland (right) or perirenal and/or renal sinus fat (left) but not beyond Gerota's fascia.

T3b

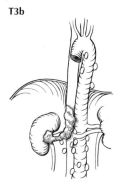

FIGURE 36.7. T3b: tumor grossly extends into the renal vein or its segmental (muscle-containing) branches, or vena cava below the diaphragm.

T3b   Tumor grossly extends into the renal vein or its segmental (muscle-containing) branches, or vena cava below the diaphragm (Figure 36.7)

T3c   Tumor grossly extends into vena cava above diaphragm or invades the wall of the vena cava (Figure 36.8)

T4   Tumor invades beyond Gerota's fascia (Figure 36.9)

Regional Lymph Nodes (N)

NX   Regional lymph nodes cannot be assessed
N0   No regional lymph node metastases
N1   Metastasis in a single regional lymph node (Figure 36.10)
N2   Metastasis in more than one regional lymph node (Figures 36.10, 36.11)

Distant Metastasis (M)

MX   Distant metastasis cannot be assessed
M0   No distant metastasis
M1   Distant metastasis

T3c

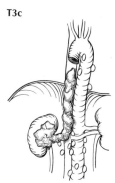

FIGURE 36.8. T3c: tumor grossly extends into vena cava above diaphragm or invades the wall of the vena cava.

36

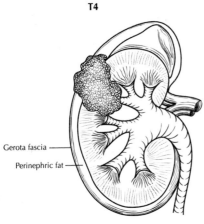

T4

FIGURE 36.9. T4: tumor invades beyond Gerota's fascia.

Gerota fascia

Perinephric fat

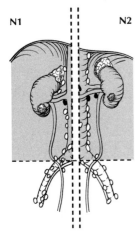

N1   N2

FIGURE 36.10. N1, on the left, is defined as metastasis in a single regional lymph node. N2, on the right, is defined as metastasis in more than one regional lymph node.

N2

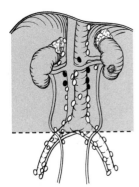

FIGURE 36.11. N2: Metastasis in more than one regional lymph node.

STAGE GROUPING

I	T1	N0	M0
II	T2	N0	M0
III	T1	N1	M0
	T2	N1	M0
	T3	N0	M0
	T3	N1	M0
	T3a	N0	M0
	T3a	N1	M0
	T3b	N0	M0
	T3b	N1	M0
	T3c	N0	M0
	T3c	N1	M0
IV	T4	N0	M0
	T4	N1	M0
	Any T	N2	M0
	Any T	Any N	M1

36

37

Renal Pelvis and Ureter

C65.9   Renal pelvis   C66.9   Ureter

SUMMARY OF CHANGES

• The definitions of TNM and the Stage Grouping for this chapter have not changed from the Fifth Edition.

INTRODUCTION

Urothelial (transitional cell) carcinoma may occur at any site within the upper urinary collecting system from the renal calyx to the ureterovesical junction. The tumors occur most commonly in adults and are rare before 40 years of age. There is a two- to threefold increase in incidence in men compared with women. The lesions are often multiple and are more common in patients with a history of urothelial carcinoma of the bladder. A number of analgesics (such as phenacetin) have also been associated with this disease. Local staging depends on the depth of invasion. A common staging system is used regardless of tumor location within the upper urinary collecting system, except for category T3, which differs between the pelvis or calyceal system and the ureter.

ANATOMY

Primary Site. The renal pelvis and the ureter form a single unit that is continuous with the collecting ducts of the renal pyramids and comprises the minor and major calyces, which are continuous with the renal pelvis. The ureteropelvic junction is variable in position and location but serves as a "landmark" that separates the renal pelvis and the ureter, which continues caudad and traverses the wall of the urinary bladder as the intramural ureter opening in the trigone of the bladder at the ureteral orifice. The renal pelvis and the ureter are composed of the following layers: epithelium, subepithelial connective tissue, and muscularis, which is continuous with a connective tissue adventitial layer. It is in this outer layer that the major blood supply and lymphatics are found.

The intrarenal portion of the renal pelvis is surrounded by renal parenchyma, and the extrarenal pelvis by perihilar fat. The ureter courses through the retroperitoneum adjacent to the parietal peritoneum and rests on the retroperitoneal musculature above the pelvic vessels. As it crosses the vessels and enters the deep pelvis, the ureter is surrounded by pelvic fat until it traverses the bladder wall.

Regional Lymph Nodes. The regional lymph nodes for the renal pelvis are:

Renal hilar
Paracaval
Aortic
Retroperitoneal, NOS

The regional lymph nodes for the ureter are:

Renal hilar
Iliac (common, internal [hypogastric], external)
Paracaval
Periureteral
Pelvic, NOS

Any amount of regional lymph node metastasis is a poor prognostic finding and outcome is minimally influenced by the number, size, or location of the regional nodes that are involved.

Metastatic Sites. Distant spread is most commonly to the lung, bone, or liver.

DEFINITIONS

Primary Tumor (T)

TX	Primary tumor cannot be assessed
T0	No evidence of primary tumor
Ta	Papillary noninvasive carcinoma (Figure 37.1)
Tis	Carcinoma *in situ*
T1	Tumor invades subepithelial connective tissue (Figure 37.1)
T2	Tumor invades the muscularis (Figure 37.2)
T3	(For renal pelvis only) Tumor invades beyond muscularis into peripelvic fat or the renal parenchyma (Figure 37.2)
T3	(For ureter only) Tumor invades beyond muscularis into periureteric fat
T4	Tumor invades adjacent organs, or through the kidney into the perinephric fat (Figures 37.3A–C)

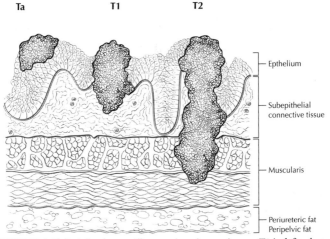

FIGURE 37.1. Ta is defined as papillary noninvasive carcinoma; T1 is defined as tumor invading subepithelial connective tissue; T2 is defined as tumor invading the muscularis.

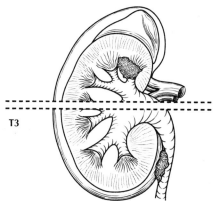

T3

T3

FIGURE 37.2. T3 (for renal pelvis only, top of diagram): tumor invades beyond muscularis into peripelvic fat or the renal parenchyma. T3 (for ureter only, bottom of diagram): tumor invades beyond muscularis into periureteric fat.

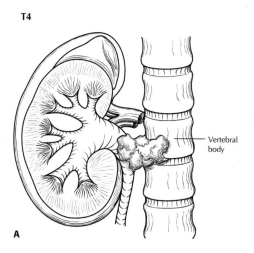

T4

Vertebral body

A

FIGURE 37.3. A. T4 tumor invades adjacent organs, or through the kidney into the perinephric fat. Here, the tumor invades the vertebral body.

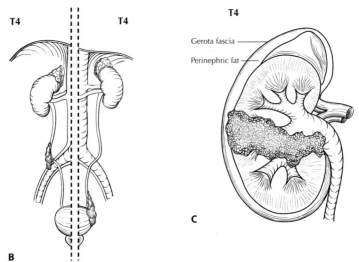

FIGURE 37.3. B. T4 tumor (ureter) invades adjacent organs. On the left, tumor invades the iliac vessels. On the right, tumor invades the bladder. **C.** T4 tumor invades through the kidney into the perinephric fat.

Regional Lymph Nodes (N)

NX Regional lymph nodes cannot be assessed

N0 No regional lymph node metastasis

N1 Metastasis in a single lymph node, 2 cm or less in greatest dimension (Figure 37.4)

N2 Metastasis in a single lymph node, more than 2 cm but not more than 5 cm in greatest dimension; or multiple lymph nodes, none more than 5 cm in greatest dimension (Figures 37.5A, B)

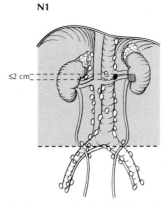

FIGURE 37.4. N1 is defined as metastasis in a single lymph node, 2 cm or less in greatest dimension.

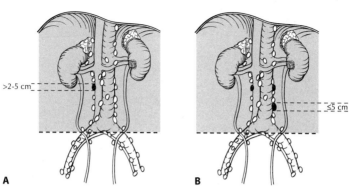

FIGURE 37.5. A. N2 nodal metastasis in a single lymph node, more than 2 cm but not more than 5 cm in greatest dimension, as illustrated; or multiple lymph nodes, none more than 5 cm in greatest dimension **B.** N2 nodal metastasis in a single lymph node, more than 2 cm but not more than 5 cm in greatest dimension; or multiple lymph nodes, none more than 5 cm in greatest dimension, as illustrated.

N3   Metastasis in a lymph node, more than 5 cm in greatest dimension (Figures 37.6A, B)

Distant Metastasis (M)

MX   Distant metastasis cannot be assessed
M0   No distant metastasis
M1   Distant metastasis

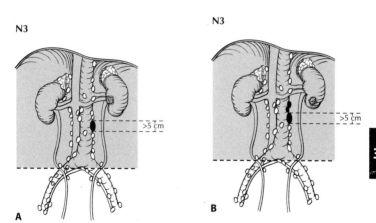

FIGURE 37.6. A. N3 is defined as metastasis in a lymph node, more than 5 cm in greatest dimension. **B.** N3 nodal metastasis in a lymph node, more than 5 cm in greatest dimension. As illustrated here, multiple lymph nodes are involved with one nodal mass exceeding 5 cm.

STAGE GROUPING

0a	Ta	N0	M0
0is	Tis	N0	M0
I	T1	N0	M0
II	T2	N0	M0
III	T3	N0	M0
IV	T4	N0	M0
	Any T	N1	M0
	Any T	N2	M0
	Any T	N3	M0
	Any T	Any N	M1

C67.0	Trigone of bladder	C67.4	Posterior wall of	C67.8	Overlapping lesion of
C67.1	Dome of bladder		bladder		bladder
C67.2	Lateral wall of	C67.5	Bladder neck	C67.9	Bladder, NOS
	bladder	C67.6	Ureteric orifice		
C67.3	Anterior wall of	C67.7	Urachus		
	bladder				

SUMMARY OF CHANGES
- The definitions of TNM and the Stage Grouping for this chapter have not changed from the Fifth Edition.

INTRODUCTION

Bladder cancer is one of the most common malignancies in Western society, and it occurs more commonly in males. Predisposing factors include smoking, exposure to chemicals, such as phenacetin and dyes, and schistosomiasis. It has also been suggested that the incidence of this disease correlates inversely with fluid intake. Hematuria is the most common presenting feature. Bladder cancer can present as a low-grade papillary lesion, as an *in situ* lesion that can occupy large areas of the mucosal surface, or as an infiltrative cancer that rapidly extends through the bladder wall and can thereafter metastasize. The papillary and *in situ* lesions may be associated with a malignant course, with sudden invasion of the bladder wall. The most common histologic variant is urothelial (transitional cell) carcinomas, although this may exhibit features of glandular or squamous differentiation. In less than 10% of cases, pure adenocarcinoma or squamous carcinoma of the bladder may occur, and less frequently, sarcoma, lymphoma, small cell anaplastic carcinoma, pheochromocytoma, choriocarcinoma. Squamous carcinoma is associated with schistosomiasis and smoking.

ANATOMY

Primary Site. The anatomic sites and subsites of the urinary bladder are illustrated in Figure 38.1. The urinary bladder consists of three layers: the epithelium and the subepithelial connective tissue, the muscularis, and the perivesical fat (peritoneum covering the superior surface and upper part). In the male, the bladder adjoins the rectum and seminal vesicle posteriorly, the prostate inferiorly, and the pubis and peritoneum anteriorly. In the female, the vagina is located posteriorly and the uterus superiorly. The bladder is located extraperitoneally.

Regional Lymph Nodes. The regional lymph nodes are the nodes of the true pelvis (Figure 38.2), which essentially are the pelvic nodes below the bifurcation of the common iliac arteries. The significance of regional lymph node metastasis in staging bladder cancer lies in the number and size, not in whether metastasis is unilateral or contralateral. One of the major prognostic determinants of

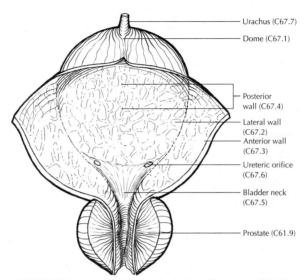

FIGURE 38.1. Anatomical sites and subsites of the urinary bladder.

ultimate cure is whether the tumor is confined to the bladder, and a major adverse prognostic feature is the presence of *any* lymph nodal metastases.

Regional nodes include:

Hypogastric
Obturator

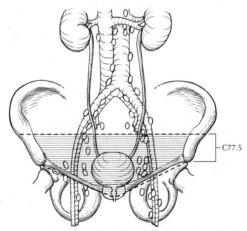

FIGURE 38.2. Regional lymph nodes of the urinary bladder.

Iliac (internal, external, NOS)
Perivesical
Pelvic, NOS
Sacral (lateral, sacral promontory [Gerota's])
Presacral

The common iliac nodes are considered sites of distant metastasis and should be coded as M1.

Metastatic Sites. Distant spread is most commonly to lymph nodes, lung, bone, and liver.

DEFINITIONS

Primary Tumor (T)

TX   Primary tumor cannot be assessed
T0   No evidence of primary tumor
Ta   Noninvasive papillary carcinoma (Figure 38.3)
Tis Carcinoma *in situ*: "flat tumor" (Figure 38.3)
T1   Tumor invades subepithelial connective tissue (Figure 38.3)
T2   Tumor invades muscle (Figure 38.3)

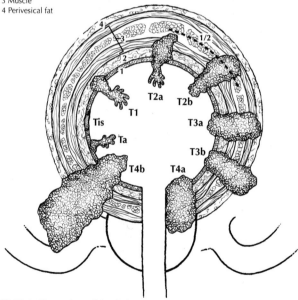

1 Epithelium
2 Subepithelial connective tissue
3 Muscle
4 Perivesical fat

FIGURE 38.3. Illustration of the definitions of primary tumor (T) for primary bladder cancer, ranging from Ta to T4.

pT2a	Tumor invades superficial muscle (inner half)
pT2b	Tumor invades deep muscle (outer half)
T3	Tumor invades perivesical tissue (Figure 38.3)
pT3a	Microscopically
pT3b	Macroscopically (extravesical mass)
T4	Tumor invades any of the following: prostate, uterus, vagina, pelvic wall, abdominal wall
T4a	Tumor invades prostate, uterus, vagina (Figure 38.3)
T4b	Tumor invades pelvic wall, abdominal wall (Figure 38.3)

Regional Lymph Nodes (N)

NX   Regional lymph nodes cannot be assessed

N0   No regional lymph node metastasis

Nl   Metastasis in a single lymph node, 2 cm or less in greatest dimension (Figure 38.4)

N2   Metastasis in a single lymph node, more than 2 cm but not more than 5 cm in greatest dimension; or multiple lymph nodes, none more than 5 cm in greatest dimension (Figures 38.5A, B)

N3   Metastasis in a lymph node, more than 5 cm in greatest dimension (Figures 38.6A, B)

Distant Metastasis (M)

MX   Distant metastasis cannot be assessed

M0   No distant metastasis

M1   Distant metastasis

N1

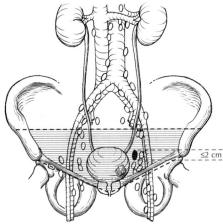

FIGURE 38.4. N1 is defined as metastasis in a single lymph node, 2 cm or less in greatest dimension.

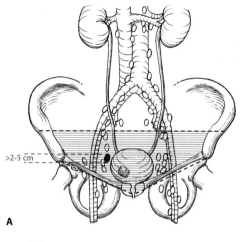

>2-5 cm

A

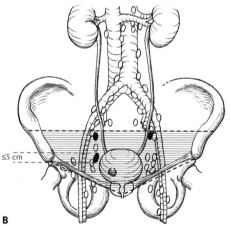

≤5 cm

B

FIGURE 38.5. A. N2 is defined as metastasis in a single lymph node, more than 2 cm but not more than 5 cm in greatest dimension, as illustrated, or multiple lymph nodes, none more than 5 cm in greatest dimension. **B.** N2 is defined as metastasis in a single lymph node, more than 2 cm but not more than 5 cm in greatest dimension, or multiple lymph nodes, as illustrated, none more than 5 cm in greatest dimension.

38

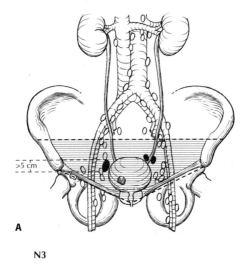

N3

FIGURE 38.6. A. N3 is defined as metastasis in a lymph node more than 5 cm in greatest dimension. Here, multiple lymph nodes are involved with one nodal mass greater than 5 cm. **B.** N3 is defined as metastasis in a lymph node more than 5 cm in greatest dimension.

STAGE GROUPING

0a	Ta	N0	M0
0is	Tis	N0	M0
I	T1	N0	M0
II	T2a	N0	M0
	T2b	N0	M0
III	T3a	N0	M0
	T3b	N0	M0
	T4a	N0	M0
IV	T4b	N0	M0
	Any T	Nl	M0
	Any T	N2	M0
	Any T	N3	M0
	Any T	Any N	M1

38

39

Urethra

C68.0   Urethra

SUMMARY OF CHANGES

• The definitions of TNM and the Stage Grouping for this chapter have not changed from the Fifth Edition.

INTRODUCTION

Cancer of the urethra is a rare neoplasia that is found in both sexes but is more common in females. The cancer may be associated in males with chronic stricture disease and in females with urethral diverticula. Tumors of the urethra may be of primary origin from the urethral epithelium or ducts, or they may be associated with multifocal urothelial neoplasia. Histologically, these tumors may represent the spectrum of epithelial neoplasms, including squamous, adenothelial, or urothelial (transitional cell) carcinoma. Prostatic urethral neoplasms arising from the prostatic urethral epithelium or from the periurethral portion of the prostatic ducts are considered urethral neoplasms as distinct from those arising elsewhere in the prostate (see Chapter 34).

ANATOMY

Primary Site. The male urethra consists of mucosa, submucosal stroma, and the surrounding corpus spongiosum. Histologically, the meatal and parameatal urethra are lined with squamous cell epithelium, the penile and bulbomembranous urethra with pseudostratified or stratified columnar epithelium, and bulbomembranithelium, and the prostatic urethra with transitional epithelium. There are scattered islands of stratified squamous epithelium and glands of Littré liberally situated throughout the entire urethra distal to the prostate portion.

The epithelium of the female urethra is supported on subepithelial connective tissue. The periurethral glands of Skene are concentrated near the meatus but extend along the entire urethra. The urethra is surrounded by a longitudinal layer of smooth muscle continuous with the bladder. The urethra is contiguous to the vaginal wall. The distal two-thirds of the urethra is lined with squamous epithelium, the proximal one-third with transitional epithelium. The periurethral glands are lined with pseduostratified and stratified columnar epithelium.

Regional Lymph Nodes. The regional lymph nodes are:

Inguinal (superficial or deep)
Iliac (common, internal [hypogastric], obturator, external)
Presacral
Sacral, NOS
Pelvic, NOS

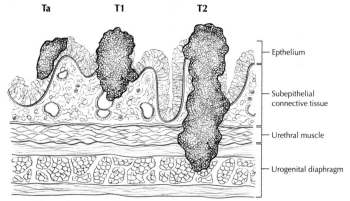

FIGURE 39.1. Illustrated definitions of primary tumor (T) for Ta, T1, and T2 with depth of invasion ranging from the epithelium to the urogenital diaphragm.

The significance of regional lymph node metastasis in staging urethral cancer lies in the number and size, not in whether unilateral or bilateral.

Metastatic Sites. Distant spread is most commonly to lung, liver, or bone.

DEFINITIONS

Primary Tumor (T)
(Male and Female)

TX Primary tumor cannot be assessed

T0 No evidence of primary tumor

Ta Noninvasive papillary, polypoid, or verrucous carcinoma (Figures 39.1, 39.2)

Tis Carcinoma *in situ*

T1 Tumor invades subepithelial connective tissue (Figures 39.1, 39.3)

T2 Tumor invades any of the following: corpus spongiosum, prostate, periurethral muscle (Figures 39.1, 39.4, 39.5)

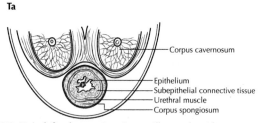

FIGURE 39.2. Ta is defined as noninvasive papillary, polypoid, or verrucous carcinoma.

T1

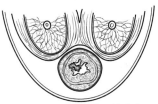

FIGURE 39.3. T1 tumor invading subepithelial connective tissue.

T2

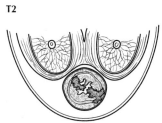

FIGURE 39.4. T2 tumor invades any of the following: corpus spongiosum, prostate, periurethral muscle (as illustrated).

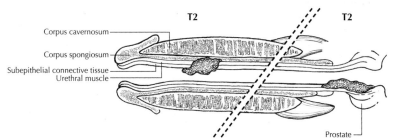

FIGURE 39.5. Two views of T2 tumor in the male with invasion of the corpus spongiosum (left) and the prostate (right).

T3   Tumor invades any of the following: corpus cavernosum, beyond prostatic capsule, anterior vagina, bladder neck (Figures 39.6A–C)

T4   Tumor invades other adjacent organs (Figure 39.7)

Urothelial (Transitional Cell) Carcinoma of the Prostate

Tis pu   Carcinoma *in situ,* involvement of the prostatic urethra (Figure 39.8A)

Tis pd   Carcinoma *in situ,* involvement of the prostatic ducts (Figure 39.8B)

T1   Tumor invades subepithelial connective tissue (Figures 39.8A, B)

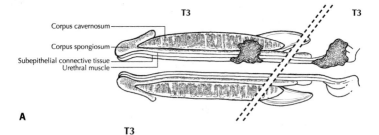

A

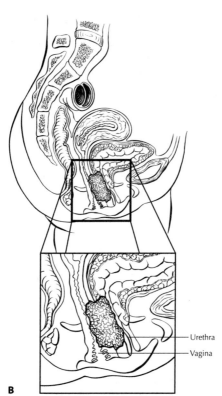

B

FIGURE 39.6. A. Two views of T3 tumor in the male with invasion of the corpus cavernosum (left) and prostatic capsule (right). **B.** T3 tumor in the female with invasion of the anterior vagina.

T3

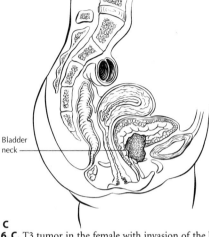

Bladder neck

C

FIGURE 39.6. C. T3 tumor in the female with invasion of the bladder neck.

T4

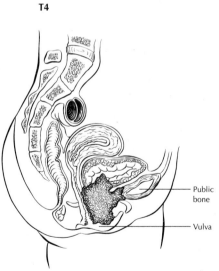

Public bone

Vulva

FIGURE 39.7. T4 tumor in the female with invasion to other adjacent organs (here, the pubic bone and vulva).

39

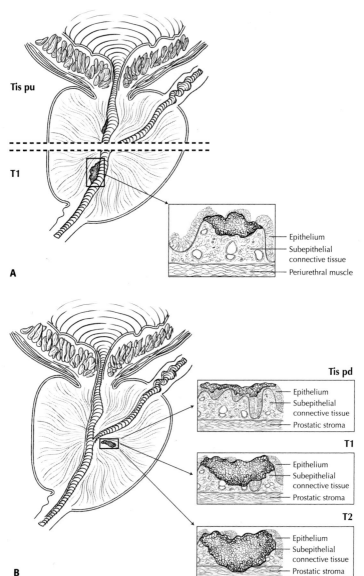

FIGURE 39.8. A. The definition of Tis pu for urothelial (transitional cell) carcinoma of the prostate (above dotted lines) is carcinoma *in situ,* involvement of the prostatic urethra. T1 (below dotted lines) is defined as tumor invading subepithelial connective tissue. **B.** Definitions of primary tumor (T) for urothelial (transitional cell) carcinoma of the prostate for Tis pd, T1, and T2 with depth of invasion ranging from the epithelium to the prostatic stroma.

T2

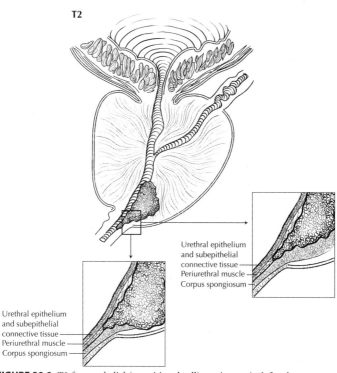

Urethral epithelium
and subepithelial
connective tissue
Periurethral muscle
Corpus spongiosum

Urethral epithelium
and subepithelial
connective tissue
Periurethral muscle
Corpus spongiosum

FIGURE 39.9. T2 for urothelial (transitional cell) carcinoma is defined as tumor invading any of the following: prostatic stroma, corpus spongiosum, periurethral muscle.

T2   Tumor invades any of the following: prostatic stroma, corpus spongiosum, periurethral muscle (Figures 39.8B, 39.9)

T3   Tumor invades any of the following: corpus cavernosum, beyond prostatic capsule, bladder neck (extraprostatic extension) (Figure 39.10)

T4   Tumor invades other adjacent organs (invasion of the bladder) (Figure 39.11)

Regional Lymph Nodes (N)

NX   Regional lymph nodes cannot be assessed

N0   No regional lymph node metastasis

N1   Metastasis in a single lymph node 2 cm or less in greatest dimension (Figure 39.12)

N2   Metastasis in a single node more than 2 cm in greatest dimension, or in multiple nodes (Figures 39.13A, B)

Distant Metastasis (M)

MX   Distant metastasis cannot be assessed

M0   No distant metastasis

M1   Distant metastasis

39

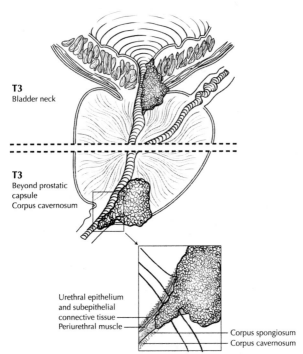

FIGURE 39.10. Two views of T3 for urothelial (transitional cell) carcinoma. Tumor invades any of the following: corpus cavernosum, as illustrated below dotted lines; beyond prostatic capsule; bladder neck (extraprostatic extension), as illustrated above dotted lines.

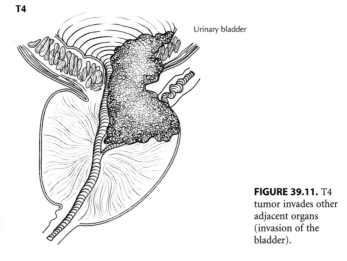

FIGURE 39.11. T4 tumor invades other adjacent organs (invasion of the bladder).

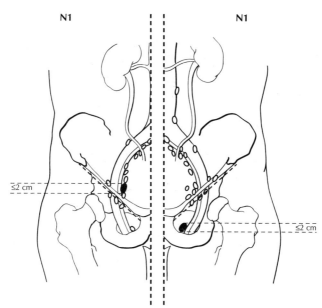

FIGURE 39.12. N1 is defined as metastasis in a single lymph node 2 cm or less in greatest dimension.

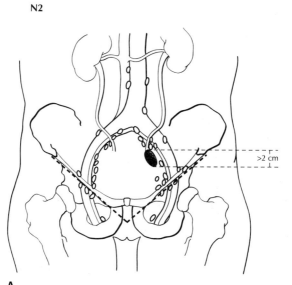

A

FIGURE 39.13. A. N2 is defined as metastasis in a single node more than 2 cm in greatest dimension, as illustrated, or in multiple nodes.

39

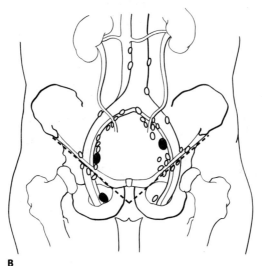

B

FIGURE 39.13. B. N2 is defined as metastasis in a single node more than 2 cm in greatest dimension or in multiple nodes, as illustrated.

STAGE GROUPING

0a	Ta	N0	M0
0is	Tis	N0	M0
	Tis pu	N0	M0
	Tis pd	N0	M0
I	T1	N0	M0
II	T2	N0	M0
III	T1	N1	M0
	T2	N1	M0
	T3	N0	M0
	T3	N1	M0
IV	T4	N0	M0
	T4	N1	M0
	Any T	N2	M0
	Any T	Any N	M1

Index

regional lymph nodes (N)
  classification, 181
risk factors, 177
stage grouping, 181–182
staging systems for, 177–178
Prefix descriptors, 8
Pregnancy. *See* Gestational
  trophoblastic tumors
Primary tumor (T)
  definitions, 7
  notations used, 7
Prostate, 293–301
  distant lymph nodes, 295
  distant metastasis (M), 300
  histologic grade (G), 300
  metastatic sites, 295
  pathologic (pT), 297
  primary site, 293–294
  primary tumor (T), 295–298
  regional lymph nodes, 294
  regional lymph nodes (N)
    classification, 299–300
  regional lymph nodes (pN)
    classification, 300
  stage grouping, 300

R

Rectum
  anatomical subsites, 108–109
  See also Colon and rectum
Regional lymph nodes (N)
  definitions, 7
  notations used, 7
Renal pelvis and ureter, 323–328
  distant metastasis (M), 327
  metastatic sites, 324
  primary site, 323
  primary tumor (T), 324–326
  regional lymph nodes, 323–324
  regional lymph nodes (N)
    classification, 326–327
  stage grouping, 328
Residual tumor, notation used, 9
Retreatment classification, elements of,
  6
Retromolar gingiva
  features/location, 21
  See also Lips and oral cavity
r prefix, meaning of, 8

S

Salivary glands, 61–66
  distant metastasis (M), 65
  metastatic sites, 62
  primary site, 61

primary tumor (T), 62–65
  regional lymph nodes, 61–62
  regional lymph nodes (N)
    classification, 65
  stage grouping, 66
Sarcomas. *See* Soft tissue sarcomas
Sinuses, paranasal. *See* Nasal cavity and
  paranasal sinuses
Skin. *See* Carcinoma of the skin;
  Melanoma of the skin
Small intestine, 101–106
  distant metastasis (M), 106
  duodenum, 101, 102–103
  ileum, 102, 103
  jejunum, 102, 103
  metastatic sites, 103
  primary sites, 101–102
  primary tumor (T), 103–106
  regional lymph nodes, 102–103
  regional lymph nodes (N)
    classification, 106
  stage grouping, 106
Soft tissue sarcoma, 191–194
  distant metastasis (M), 194
  histologic grade (G), 192, 194
  inclusions, 192
  metastatic sites, 192–193
  primary tumor (T), 193–194
  regional lymph nodes, 192
  regional lymph nodes (N)
    classification, 194
  site groups for sarcomas, 192
  stage grouping, 194
Stage grouping
  functions of, 9
  stages, meaning of, 9
Staging, general rules, 3–4
Stomach, 89–99
  distant metastasis (M), 92
  metastatic sites, 92
  primary site, 90–91
  primary tumor (T), 92–96
  regional lymph nodes, 91–92
  regional lymph nodes (N)
    classification, 92, 97–98
  stage grouping, 99
Subglottis
  features/location, 41–42
  primary tumor, 49–50
  See also Larynx
Sublingual gland. *See* Salivary
  glands
Submandibular gland. *See* Salivary
  glands
Suffix descriptors, 8